D1552383

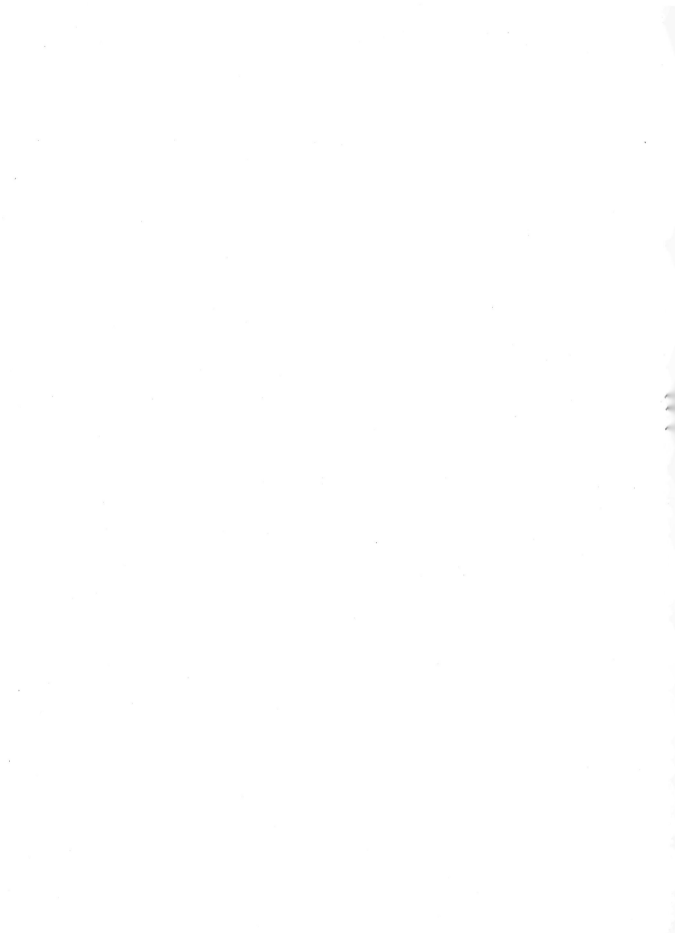

Practical Phlebology

Venous
Ultrasound

Practical Phlebology

Series Editors: Lowell S Kabnick, Neil S Sadick

PUBLISHED

Practical Phlebology: Starting and Managing a Phlebology Practice
Marlin Schul; Saundra Spruiell; Clint Hayes
2010 • ISBN 9781853159404

Practical Phlebology: Venous Ultrasound
Joseph Zygmunt; Olivier Pichot; Tracie Dauplaise
2013 • ISBN 9781853159404

FORTHCOMING
Practical Phlebology: Deep Vein Thrombosis
Anthony J. Comerota
ISBN 9781444146097

Practical Phlebology

Venous Ultrasound

Joseph Zygmunt Jr, Olivier Pichot,
Tracie Dauplaise

Series Editors:
Lowell Kabnick MD FACS Associate Professor
of Surgery, New York University,
Langone Medical Center, New York; and
Director, NYU Vein Center, NY, USA
Neil Sadick MD FAAD FAACS FACPH
Clinical Professor of Dermatology,
Weill Cornell Medical College,
Cornell University, New York, NY, USA

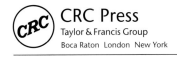

CRC Press
Taylor & Francis Group
Boca Raton London New York

CRC Press is an imprint of the
Taylor & Francis Group, an **informa** business

CRC Press
Taylor & Francis Group
6000 Broken Sound Parkway NW, Suite 300
Boca Raton, FL 33487-2742

© 2013 by Taylor & Francis Group, LLC
CRC Press is an imprint of Taylor & Francis Group, an Informa business

No claim to original U.S. Government works

Printed on acid-free paper
Version Date: 20130412

Printed and bound in India by Replika Press Pvt. Ltd.

International Standard Book Number-13: 978-1-85315-948-0 (Hardback)

This book contains information obtained from authentic and highly regarded sources. While all reasonable efforts have been made to publish reliable data and information, neither the author[s] nor the publisher can accept any legal responsibility or liability for any errors or omissions that may be made. The publishers wish to make clear that any views or opinions expressed in this book by individual editors, authors or contributors are personal to them and do not necessarily reflect the views/opinions of the publishers. The information or guidance contained in this book is intended for use by medical, scientific or health-care professionals and is provided strictly as a supplement to the medical or other professional's own judgement, their knowledge of the patient's medical history, relevant manufacturer's instructions and the appropriate best practice guidelines. Because of the rapid advances in medical science, any information or advice on dosages, procedures or diagnoses should be independently verified. The reader is strongly urged to consult the drug companies' printed instructions, and their websites, before administering any of the drugs recommended in this book. This book does not indicate whether a particular treatment is appropriate or suitable for a particular individual. Ultimately it is the sole responsibility of the medical professional to make his or her own professional judgements, so as to advise and treat patients appropriately. The authors and publishers have also attempted to trace the copyright holders of all material reproduced in this publication and apologize to copyright holders if permission to publish in this form has not been obtained. If any copyright material has not been acknowledged please write and let us know so we may rectify in any future reprint.

Except as permitted under U.S. Copyright Law, no part of this book may be reprinted, reproduced, transmitted, or utilized in any form by any electronic, mechanical, or other means, now known or hereafter invented, including photocopying, microfilming, and recording, or in any information storage or retrieval system, without written permission from the publishers.

For permission to photocopy or use material electronically from this work, please access www.copyright.com (http://www.copyright.com/) or contact the Copyright Clearance Center, Inc. (CCC), 222 Rosewood Drive, Danvers, MA 01923, 978-750-8400. CCC is a not-for-profit organization that provides licenses and registration for a variety of users. For organizations that have been granted a photocopy license by the CCC, a separate system of payment has been arranged.

Trademark Notice: Product or corporate names may be trademarks or registered trademarks, and are used only for identification and explanation without intent to infringe.

**Visit the Taylor & Francis Web site at
http://www.taylorandfrancis.com**

**and the CRC Press Web site at
http://www.crcpress.com**

Dedication

What influences the development of a person? Imitation and/or emulation is the highest form of respect and, yes, flattery. To live one's life and 'always do the right thing' can sometimes be a long hard road, yet this was instilled at a very young age. Recently, I heard the quote 'no deposit–no return' and although this quote is new to me, it resonated to the very core of my being. Without knowing it, this was really the lesson learned from my parents, Eleanor and Joe. Eleanor and Joe were each first-generation offspring of immigrants from Krakow, Poland. During their younger years, they were tasked with teaching English to their parents and grandparents after school as they grew up in a coal mining town of Northeast Pennsylvania.

Dad entered the military and, upon returning home, married the hometown girl who lived just down the road. They traveled to Idaho, South Florida, and Massachusetts before settling just outside Philadelphia to the only home I've ever known. A 30+ year employee of Boeing, Dad provided for us, completed his college education later in life, while Mom was the consummate mother and housekeeper in every traditional sense. The lessons we learned – seemingly like the 'paint the fence' maneuver from Karate Kid, proved to be the most significant in grounding a work ethic, kindness, generosity, and moral integrity that has served my siblings and me unendingly. The love, personal sacrifice, and support was limitless, and for that I (we) am eternally grateful. I would thank you from the bottom of my heart, but for you my heart has no bottom.

So great was the respect and admiration Eleanor and Joe had for the medical establishment that all four of their children wound up in the fields of pharmacy, nursing, or phlebology. The oldest of the grandchildren also has a PharmD, and the remaining grandchildren, just in elementary school, have a few years left to decide on a career path.

Catch phrases like 'always do the right thing' serve as the basis and constant reminder that *we get what we give* and *we can do better*. And so in conclusion, I am amazingly grateful to Eleanor and Joe as they've instilled in their children goals to *reach for the stars* and *aspire to be the best that we can* – period!

Joe Zygmunt Jr

Don't bother just to be better than your contemporaries or predecessors.
Try to be better than yourself.

William Faulkner

Rule #1: Use your good judgment in all situations. There will be no additional rules.

Nordstrom's Employee Handbook

The most important human endeavor is striving for morality in our actions. Our inner balance and even our very existence depend on it. Only morality in our actions can give beauty and dignity to our lives.

Albert Einstein

My grandfather once told me that there are two kinds of people: those who work and those who take the credit. He told me to try to be in the first group; there was less competition there.

Indira Gandhi

Let parents bequeath to their children not riches, but the spirit of reverence.

Plato

I'll tell you a big secret, my friend: Don't wait for the Last Judgment. It happens every day.

Albert Camus

Contents

Foreword

It is with great enthusiasm and fortitude that I introduce the second manual of the Practical Phlebology series: *Venous Ultrasound*. The first release entitled, *Starting and Managing a Phlebology Practice*, was written by Marlin Schul, Saundra Spruiell, and Clint Hayes.

The series of Practical Phlebology would be remiss not to include one of the most important components regarding diagnosis and treatment of venous disease: ultrasound. Ultrasound has become an integral part of phlebology providing the modernization of both diagnosis and treatment. Presently, the use of ultrasound has facilitated the development of minimally invasive venous procedures and all the inherent benefits. Prior to this imaging modality, the diagnosis of superficial reflux, deep vein reflux, and DVT was based on clinical findings. Before procedural ultrasound became the standard of care, venous intervention was blind. Many patients were treated incorrectly and some suffered complications.

We are extremely fortunate to have as the author of *Venous Ultrasound*, Joseph Zygmut Jr RVT, RPhS with co-authors, Tracie Dauplaise RVT, RPhS and Olivier Pichot MD. One of the most challenging aspects in the diagnosis of venous disease is the performance and understanding of venous duplex. These authors have been instrumental in the education of many physicians and technologists. Hopefully, you will benefit from their hard work, as have I.

Lowell Kabnick

Preface

The phlebology practice has grown tremendously in the last decade. Many specialists from different disciplines, such as vascular, general, cardiothoracic and plastic surgery, internal and vascular medicine, interventional radiology, cardiology, family practice, and phlebology work on the diagnosis and management of chronic venous disease (CVD). Also imaging specialists, vascular technologists, physician assistants, and nurses play an integral role on the delivery of care of patients with CVD. The book on practical phlebology and venous ultrasound is a great addition in the literature due to its direct application into clinical practice and it is very useful for all the practitioners and specialists mentioned above. The authors are well known in the field of phlebology and ultrasound and have done remarkable work. The book covers many relevant topics in clinical phlebology and it is an important aid for those who are involved in the diagnosis and management of CVD. The book has reasonable size with 160 pages containing the most useful topics for understanding ultrasound and its application before, during, and after treatment. It contains nine sections filled with information that mostly focuses on clinical practice without deviating into long explanations on theories and mechanisms of disease. Many tips and tricks have been inserted with more emphasis to enhance the understanding and importance of the knowledge provided in each chapter. This is invaluable information as many simple and complex concepts and themes are given in a practical manner in order to facilitate the application of ultrasound and treatment modalities used in patients with CVD. It has great illustrations with detailed information on important imaging and treating aspects of CVD. The ultrasound images are of high quality demonstrating venous anatomy and variations together with the surrounding tissues and all aspects of pathology. Excellent diagrams, figures, and tables complement the images and the text to give a comprehensive understanding of each subject. The book appropriately has half of its content covered by illustrations. The combination of the simple and clear diagrams and ultrasound images provide a very good understanding of the anatomy and pathology of the venous system and of the imaging techniques in amalgamation with the patient treatment and follow up. A great example here is the detailed demonstration of how to get vein access with ultrasound guidance. Many tips and tricks are given and full explanation with text, diagrams, and images are provided to allow great understanding of this simple technique which is vital in performing endovenous treatment in the everyday practice. In addition, the protocols of examination take this a step further as they allow proper patient evaluation and aid in the streamlining of the work flow. In summary, this is a great practical illustrated guide on the phlebology practice that will be very useful for the trainees and all of those who perform diagnosis and treatment of CVD.

Nicos Labropoulos

Acknowledgments

It can be difficult to recognize all those individuals who have had an impact in one way or another on the development of this text, or better said the professional education that led to this text. In brief, I would like to express my sincere gratitude to my co-authors, Tracie Dauplaise and Olivier Pichot, for their contributions, and hours of work on this project, Dr Lowell Kabnick, who presented me with this opportunity, and whose patience and guidance in the process, was critical. And, of course, Susie Bond, without whom the copy revision process would have been much more difficult as she helped keep us on course in so many ways.

I would also like to recognize those who have had a significant impact on my professional career and development, without whose support, guidance, and friendship the field of phlebology would not have been so comfortable for me for these many years. It is actually hard to believe that my first experience with vein therapy was with Robert Biegelisen Knight back in 1988. Following the French school of thought, Bob's traditional approach to injection sclerotherapy of the great saphenous vein and other abnormal veins, for medical as well as cosmetic therapy, was my first exposure to this niche science. We quickly embarked on a journey of ultrasound-guided sclerotherapy when he was unsuccessful with a palpation attempt to inject a partially occluded saphenofemoral junction, and said 'prove to me that the vein is still open', which I was able to do using our duplex machine. Seeing the vein with residual flow, he retrieved a needle and syringe from the next room and injected (with an iodine solution) the resistant vein under duplex guidance. We published this technique as the first US experience (1988) with duplex-guided sclerotherapy, and later learned that Michel Schadek had done so previously in France several years before.

Most profound however, was the influence, guidance, development, and brotherhood shared with John Mauriello. I like to say that 'John and I grew up' in a field that was developing during the 1990s and into the turn of the century. We started with simple injection sclerotherapy and ultrasound-guided injection of liquid sclerosants – a technique that demands the touch of a true artist – especially if that was all that was in your bag of tricks! We took on cases that were inappropriate for the traditional surgical therapy, and forged through hate mail from anonymous colleagues for our advertising and promotional activities as we grew our practice and developed our knowledge and skills. Slowly, we added ligation of the saphenous, ambulatory phlebectomy, and with the turn of the century, thermal ablation, to the litany of procedures that we used in our 'total vein care' office(s). I was with John for almost 20 years and had some of the best times learning, amassing skills and knowledge, while servicing the patients and communities in which we practiced. These experiences were unmatched and served as the foundation to a lasting friendship! Thanks, John!

The influences of colleagues, most of whom have become friends over the years, are quite numerous but a few will recognize themselves here in this list. Gratitude and appreciation is all I have and I would like to thank them immensely for sharing knowledge and friendship which will last for many years to come. Starting with Nick and Helane, these also include Steve, Mark, Diana, JJ, Attillio, Ted, Hugo, Jose, Ed, Nicos, Tony, Mark, Steve, Frank, Jeannie, Bill, Bo, Eric, Bruce, Tony, and others, all of whom are friends and respected colleagues.

Thanks one and all for sharing, growing and learning as we've moved through the amazing adventure called life!

Joe Zygmunt Jr

List of abbreviations used

AAGSV	Anterior accessory great saphenous vein	IVUS	Intravascular ultrasound
AC	Alternating current	LCD	Local coverage determination
ACP	American College of Phlebology	LRR	Light reflective rheography
ACR	American College of Radiology	MRI	Magnetic resonance imaging
ACTA	American Cardiology Technologists Association	MRV	Magnetic resonance venography
		MVO	Maximum venous outflow
AIUM	American Institute of Ultrasound in Medicine	NACT	National Alliance of Cardiovascular Technologists
AMA	American Medical Association	NBCVT	National Board of Cardiovascular Testing
APG	Air plethysmography		
ARDMS	American Registry for Diagnostic Medical Sonographers	PAGSV	Posterior accessory great saphenous vein
AVF	American Venous Forum	PASTE	Post ablation superficial thrombus extension
CCI	Cardiovascular Credentialing International	PE	Pulmonary embolism
		PEP	Pelvic escape points
CEAP	Clinical, etiologic, anatomic, pathophysiologic	PPG	Photoplethysmography
		PRF	Pulse repetition frequency
CEU	Continuing educational units	PTS	Post-thrombotic syndrome
CFA	Common femoral artery	PTV	Preterminal valve
CFV	Common femoral vein	PVs	Perforating veins
CME	Continuing medical education	PV	Popliteal vein
CPT	Current procedural terminology	PW	Pulsed wave
CT	Computed tomography	PWD	Pulsed wave Doppler
CTV	Computed tomography venography	RCIS	Registered Cardiovascular Invasive Specialist
CVD	Chronic venous disease		
CVI	Chronic venous insufficiency	RF	Radiofrequency
CW	Continuous wave	RFO	Radiofrequency endovenous obliteration
DC	Direct current		
D-PPG	Digital photoplethysmography	RPhS	Registered Phlebology Sonographer
DVT	Deep vein thrombosis	RPVI	Registered Physician in Vascular Interpretation
DVT	Deep venous thrombosis		
EF	Ejection fraction	RV	Residual volume
EHIT	Endovenous heat-induced thrombus	RVF	Residual volume fraction
ELLE	Extended long line echosclerotherapy	RVS	Registered vascular specialist
EV	Ejection volume	RVT	Registered vascular technologist
FFT	Fast Fourier transformation	SDMS	Society of Diagnostic Medical Sonography
FV	Femoral vein		
GSV	Great saphenous vein	SEPS	Subfascial endoscopic perforator surgery
Hz	Hertz		
ICAVL	Intersocietal Commission for the Accreditation of Vascular Laboratories	SEV	Superficial epigastric vein
		SFJ	Saphenofemoral junction
IPG	Impedence plethysmography	SIR	Society of Interventional Radiology
IPV	Incompetent perforating vein	SMDS	Society of Diagnostic Medical Sonography
IVC	Inferior vena cava	SPG	Strain-gauge plethysmography

SPI	Sonography Principles and Instrumentation	TV	Terminal valve
SPJ	Saphenopopliteal junction	UIP	Union Internationale de Phlébologie
SRU	Society of Radiologists in Ultrasound	US	Ultrasound
SSV	Small saphenous vein	VFI	Venous filling index
SVC	Segmental venous capacitance	VFT	Venous filling time (VFT90)
SVU	Society of Vascular Ultrasound	VRT	Venous refilling times
TE	Thigh extension	VTE	Venous thromboembolism
TGC	Time gain compensation	VV	Venous volume

An introduction to colored light?

In 1842, Christian Doppler wrote *On the Coloured Light of the Double Stars and Certain Other Stars of the Heaven*. This would be the article for which the name Doppler would become synonymous with the principle of velocity measurements, eventually leading to the development of today's Doppler-based ultrasound imaging equipment.[1]

Jumping forward considerably, venous ultrasound started with CW Doppler applications when, in 1961, Stegall and Rushmer described the first Doppler instrument and its practical application. In 1968, Sigel *et al.*[2] described a refinement of venous investigative techniques using Doppler principles. Also in 1968, Evans and Cockett, at the same time as Sumner and Strandness, described investigation of deep vein thrombosis using Doppler techniques.[3]

The introduction of venous imaging for venous diagnosis was in 1982 with a preliminary report by Steven Talbot in the journal *Bruit*.[4] After this, many others, including Drs Sumner, Strandness and Cranley, contributed greatly to the advancement of duplex ultrasound for vascular diagnosis as early pioneers. All the early work on venous diagnosis focused on the deep venous system, primarily looking for deep vein thrombosis. From a phlebology perspective, however, the true duplex revolution took place in 1984 when Dr Michel Schadeck performed the first ultrasound-guided sclerotherapy injection, which he later published in 1986.[5] This and other early papers sparked an interest in duplex investigation, the majority of which is cited in other sections of this work, but include the guidance of injections,[6] observation of the outcomes and general considerations regarding anatomic descriptions,[7-10] thus pushing our understanding of venous hemodynamics which is still unfolding today.[11-13] With the advancement in understanding in anatomy and hemodymanics, development of other more advanced treatment methodologies from catheter-directed sclerotherapy[14] to endovenous ablation and other image-guided techniques[14-18] have occurred.

REFERENCES

1. Bollinger A, Partsch H. Christian Doppler is 200 years young. *VASA* 2003; **32**: 225–33.
2. Sigel B, Popky GL, Wagner DK *et al*. Comparison of clinical and Doppler ultrasound evaluation to confirm lower extremity venous disease. *Surgery* 1968; **64**: 332–8.
3. Bergan J. *The vein book*. London: Elsevier Press, 2007.
4. Talbot SR. Use of real-time imaging in identifying deep venous obstruction: a preliminary report. *Bruit* 1982; **7**: 41–2.
5. Schadeck M. Doppler et echotomographie dans las sclerose des veines saphenes. *Phlebologie* 1986; **39**: 697–716.
6. Knight R, Vin F, Zygmunt J. 10th Congress of the International Union of Phlebologie: Ultrasonic Guidance of Injections into the Superficial Venous System, Strasbourg. 1989: 339–41.
7. Meissner M, Moneta G, Burnand K *et al*. The hemodynamics and diagnosis of venous disease. *Journal of Vascular Surgery* 2007; **46**: 4S–24S.
8. Coleridge-Smith P, Labropoulos N, Partsch H *et al*. Duplex ultrasound investigation of the veins in chronic venous disease of the lower limbs – UIP Consensus Document. Part I: Basic principles. *European Journal of Vascular and Endovascular Surgery* 2006; **31**: 83–92.
9. Cavezzi A, Labropoulos N, Partsch H *et al*. Duplex ultrasound investigation of the veins in chronic venous disease of the lower limbs – UIP Consensus Document. Part II: Anatomy. *European Journal of Vascular and Endovascular Surgery* 2006; **31**: 288–99.
10. Zygmunt J. What's new in duplex scanning of the venous system. *Perspectives in Vascular Surgery and Endovascular Therapy* 2009; **21**: 94–104.
11. Labropoulos N, Leon M, Nicolaides AN *et al*. Superficial venous insufficiency: correlation

of anatomic extent of reflux with clinical symptoms and signs. *Journal of Vascular Surgery* 2004; **40**: 953–8.

12. Labropoulos N, Leon L, Kwon S *et al.* Study of the venous reflux progression. *Journal of Vascular Surgery* 2005; **41**: 291–5.

13. Lurie F. Venous haemodynamics: what we know and don't know. *Phlebology* 2009; **24**: 3–7.

14. Parsi K. Catheter-directed sclerotherapy. *Phlebology* 2009; **24**: 98–107.

15. Kabnick LS. New horizons in the treatment of saphenous vein reflux. *Journal of Vascular Techniques* 2002; **26**: 239–46.

16. Min R, Zimmet S, Issacs M, Forrestal M. Endovenous laser treatment of the incompetent greater saphenous vein. *Journal of Vascular and Interventional Radiology* 2002; **12**: 1167–71.

17. Merchant RF, DePalma RG, Kabnick LS. Endovascular obliteration of saphenous reflux. A multicenter study. *Journal of Vascular Surgery* 2002; **35**: 729–36.

18. Dauplaise T, Weiss RA. Duplex-guided endovascular occlusion of refluxing saphenous veins. *Journal of Vascular Techniques* 2001; **25**: 79–82.

Principles of Doppler ultrasound

Basics of sound

The foundation of ultrasound is in the principles of sound and sound waves. Medical ultrasound is an extension of sonography, which was a field of study used during the Second World War when the US navy experimented with techniques in their search for submarines in the world's oceans. The key factors regarding the physics and general principles of sound waves are presented as a foundation for our understanding of venous duplex ultrasound.

Sound moves in the form of waves, i.e. sound waves. In ultrasound for medical applications, these sound waves are produced by piezoelectric crystals in the range of 2–20 MHz. The frequency of the sound wave is determined by the sound source, which is specific to the crystal. Ultrasound manufacturers take advantage of this principle to create probes of varying frequencies, allowing the investigation of various parts of the body.

For echocardiography, typical frequencies are generally 2–3 MHz (in the abdomen, 2.5–6 MHz) and for peripheral (or superficial) vascular ultrasound typical frequencies are 7.5–10 MHz. Vascular imaging probes will be described later. Transmitted sound waves obey certain principles. The parameters which are used to describe sound waves include: frequency, period, wavelength, and propagation speed (Figure 1.1).

- **Frequency**: the number of complete cycles per second
  - 1 hertz (Hz) is one cycle per second
  - Ultrasound is typically measured in MHz or 1 000 000 Hz

- **Period**: the time it takes for one cycle to occur
  - Period is also the reciprocal of frequency
- **Wavelength**: the length (distance) of one complete wave cycle
- **Propagation speed**: the speed of sound as it moves through a medium.

Sound cannot travel in a vacuum. The propagation speed of sound varies based on the medium through which it travels, and is based on its density and compressibility of the medium (Table 1.1). For soft tissue, this has been found to be an average of 1540 m/sec, which is the assumption used in most diagnostic ultrasound calculations. The speed of sound in different soft tissues varies slightly, but remains fairly close to this assumed constant. For instance, in fat, propagation speed is 1450 m/sec; in liver, blood and muscle, the speeds are 1550, 1570, 1580 m/sec, respectively.[1] In contrast, the propagation speed of sound in bone is 3500 m/sec, much different than soft tissue.[2]

> **TIP** Propagation speed is not related to frequency or amplitude of the sound waves.

Sound waves are also described using a formula that has the following three mathematically related parameters:

1) Frequency: the number of oscillations per second
2) Wavelength: the length (distance) of one complete wave cycle (Figure 1.2)
3) Speed of sound: for soft tissue, 1540 m/sec:

$$\text{Wavelength } (\lambda) = \frac{\text{speed of sound } (c)}{\text{frequency } (f)}$$

$$\lambda = c/f$$

As sound travels through a medium (soft tissue in this case), its strength is lessened over time and distance. The decrease in intensity or loss of energy is defined as 'attenuation'. There are several types of attenuation, namely reflection, scattering, absorption, and beam divergence. The attenuation is affected by two principles, frequency and the denseness of the medium. A key factor for ultrasound principles is

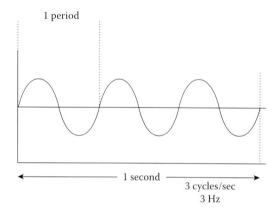

Figure 1.1 Sound wave parameters.

Table 1.1 Speed of sound in different tissue types.

Medium	Speed (m/sec)
Air	330
Water	1480
Fat	1450
Blood	1570
Muscle	1580
Bone	3500

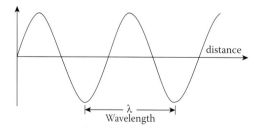

Figure 1.2 Wavelength: length (distance) of one complete wave cycle.

that attenuation is higher for higher frequencies. Therefore, a lower frequency is less attenuated than a higher one. This can also be thought of with regard to depth of penetration; a lower frequency has less attenuation and therefore can investigate a deeper structure in the body.

TIP Higher frequency ultrasound (US) probes have limited depth of penetration, so frequency and penetration are inversely proportional.

Historically, for vascular application 5.0–7.5 MHz probes are typically used for arterial and deep venous system evaluations. Probes of 7.5–10 MHz are used for superficial vein imaging. More recently, higher frequency probes of 12 and 14 MHz are being used for superficial vein mapping. Advances in technology have also produced variable frequency probes – which allow the operator to change frequency up or down depending on the depth of vessel being investigated.

In order to reduce the effects of attenuation and allow for uniform imaging, time gain compensation (TGC) is part of most ultrasound imaging systems. These do not overcome the limitations of depth and frequency penetration as noted above, but allow for uniform image quality. Figure 1.3 allows us to understand the processes that are involved in producing an ultrasound image of uniform quality and why knowledge of the TGC and slide controls impact image quality.

Another interesting fact applies directly to resolution for medical ultrasound instruments. Resolution is the ability to distinguish between two different but adjacent objects.

- Axial resolution refers to the ability to distinguish between two items along the path (or depth) of the ultrasound beam.
- Lateral resolution refers to the ability to distinguish between two items at the same depth located side by side.
- Z axis resolution, which is very important for needle visualization, and has to do with the width of the ultrasound beam.[3]

Resolution plays a key role in imaging. Figure 1.4 relates the lateral and axial resolution properties noted above. Due to the physics of the sound waves, resolution increases with higher frequencies, allowing better visualization. The 'cost' of higher resolution

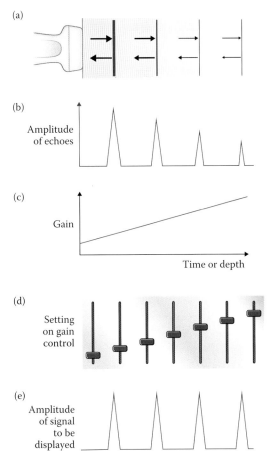

Figure 1.3 Computed time gain compensation overcome attenuation. (a) Returning echoes are weaker from more distant locations. (b) Amplitude of returning echoes. (c) Computed gain adjustment over distance and time. (d) Slide control settings as on most ultrasound machines. (e) Resulting (normalized) amplitude of returning echoes.

is less penetration (or depth). So for superficial work, there is increasing use of 12–18 MHz probes, which allows for better visualization of details such as nerves, at the cost of the deeper penetration. An adequately equipped phlebology setting should therefore consider having multiple frequency probes.

Principles of Doppler ultrasound

The principle of the Doppler or frequency shift was first published in 1842 by Austrian physicist

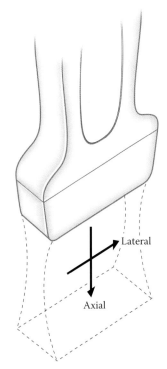

Figure 1.4 Resolution properties of the probe.

Christian Johann Doppler (Figure 1.5). Doppler hypothesized on the colored lights of the binary and certain other stars of the heavens. His theory was based on the color perceived by the eye with relation to the paired stars, and light emitted from the stars moving away from (or towards) the earth shifting its wavelength and color.

Although his hypothesis related to stars and the wavelengths of light, the basic concept was also applied to sound waves. Interestingly, in 1845, in an attempt to disprove the hypothesis, Christoph Ballot actually proved the Doppler principle, as it relates to sound waves, using musicians playing instruments on a train as it passed by. It was noticed that the frequency of the note played was perceived to increase by a semitone as the train approached, and decrease by a semitone as the train sped away.[4] This is the classic example of how sound is perceived to shift if the object is moving – in this case, the musicians on the train moved in relation to the listeners who were not moving at the station.

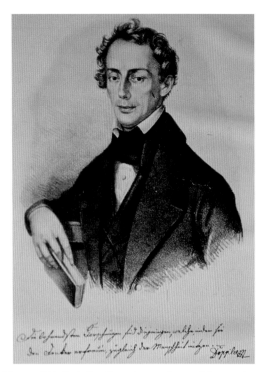

Figure 1.5 Christian Doppler, mathematician and physicist.

The Doppler effect is a result of motion, of either the source, motion of the observer, or motion of the medium, yet motion is the key factor. When it comes to analysis of blood flow, it is the motion of the blood itself which has an effect on the sound waves and resulting frequency shifts. Ultrasound instruments send and receive ultrasound waves that are bounced off moving reflectors, i.e. blood cells, resulting in a frequency shift. The difference in the frequency of the emitted and reflected sound waves is a result of the Doppler shift because of the moving blood cells. This is what we analyze and interpret to understand how the blood is flowing.

The Doppler equation expresses the relationship between several factors as noted here:

$$\Delta f = \frac{2 f_t V \cos\theta}{C} \text{ or } V = \frac{C\Delta f}{2 f_t V \cos\theta}$$

where C, average speed of sound in soft tissue (1540 m/sec); f_t, transmitted Doppler frequency; Δf, the frequency shift; $\cos\theta$, cosine theta; V, velocity (blood flow).

Piezoelectric crystals

There are crystal elements in an ultrasound transducer. These crystals are stimulated with electricity to oscillate to produce a high frequency signal (sound waves). The frequency of the transmitted signal depends on the crystal elements. The piezoelectric elements can act as both a transmitter and receiver thus allowing for emitted signals, and listening to returning sound waves which are converted back into electric energy and analyzed. The returning energy is converted and interpreted.

Also, the reflected frequencies are compared to transmitted ones and through mathematic calculations Doppler shift and blood flow velocity information is extrapolated.

Ultrasound waves

The propagation speed for sound through a medium depends on the medium itself (Table 1.2). For soft tissues in the body, this speed has been found to be about 1540 m/sec. The speed of sound is independent of the frequency and amplitude. There are several factors which affect transmission of sound. These include attenuation, refraction, and reflection. It is these factors which we take advantage of in choosing a particular frequency of ultrasound probe to insonate bodily structures of varying depths. For reinforcement of an important concept, consider the following which was previously

Table 1.2 Variable frequency probes for various body part investigations.

Frequency (MHz)	
1–4	Cardiac
1–4	Transcranial
2.5–6.6	Abdomen/pelvis
4–9	Endo (cavity)
5–10	Vascular/musculoskeletal
7.5–12	Small parts/breast
10–18	Small parts
3.5–10	Vascular
7.5–12	Vascular – phlebology
10–18	Phlebology/invasive guidance (anesthesia and others)

described. A higher frequency probe is used for superficial imaging because the higher frequency provides better resolution. Although depth is sacrificed, this is acceptable since we are looking at a superficial vessel. Using a lower frequency will allow the investigation of deeper structures. Thus, a 10+ MHz probe can be best used for saphenous imaging, while a 5 MHz probe is better for femoral (deep) vein analysis.

Continuous wave Doppler

A continuous wave (CW) Doppler instrument is comparably a very simple device, in which two separate crystals are used, one is constantly transmitting, and one is constantly receiving information, typically in a pencil probe design (Figure 1.6). The Doppler signal is audible and steerable only through the positioning or aiming of the probe. There is a constant signal emitted along a line, and the returning sound waves come from anything located along this line. This is the most significant limitation of continuous wave Doppler in that it cannot distinguish from what depth the returning sound is coming and therefore we are unable to determine if the reflux is coming from a superficial or deep venous vessel; again, the depth is unknown. One advantage is there is no aliasing artifact with continuous wave Doppler instruments. Another advantage is increased sensitivity because of the continuous signal used (versus a system in which the crystal performs both emission and reception of the signal).

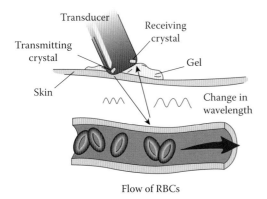

Figure 1.6 Continuous wave Doppler with separate transmit and receiving crystals.

Table 1.3 Venous flow characteristics as evaluated by Doppler.

Spontaneous	Typically in proximal veins only
Unidirectional	
Phasic	With respiration
Non-pulsatile	
Augmented	

TIP Continuous wave ultrasound does not allow for depth location. Also as there is no pulsed Doppler, there can be no aliasing artifact with CW Dopplers.

CW Doppler was once believed to be the 'stethoscope of the phlebologist'.[5] Use of a CW Doppler is a practicing art, one that is used less often with the development of duplex techniques and miniaturization of equipment.

From a historical perspective, however, it should be recognized that CW Doppler played a significant role in evaluation of the venous patient. Early diagnostic techniques relied on five venous flow characteristics,[6] which are still employed today in the era of duplex ultrasound. These flow characteristics are described in Table 1.3.

Of note, spontaneous flow is not always seen, especially in distal veins, but in more proximal segments, the lack of spontaneous flow could be indicative of flow disturbances. Augmentation maneuvers, including manual compressions proximal (deep system only) or distal to the probe, allow for interpretation of the venous flow characteristics. The learning curve for diagnosis can be quite long, and is very technique dependent. In the hands of a skilled phlebologist, much information can be obtained. Provided only for historical perspective, the next concept and figure is no longer used due to the advent of duplex ultrasound guidance. However, early on, some physicians used CW Dopplers to guide sclerosing injections before duplex guidance availability (Figure 1.7).[7, 8] Guided injections are no longer performed in this manner.

Since CW Doppler is a relatively blind investigative tool, and depths of targets are not known, one can easily mistake saphenous reflux in either the groin or popliteal fossa for deep system incompetence. The ability and access to duplex ultrasound equipment (some of which is now in laptop form)

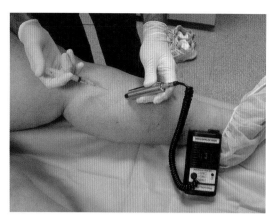

Figure 1.7 Continuous wave Doppler-guided injection. This method is no longer performed.

has all but eliminated the CW Doppler from practical everyday use in a modern phlebology office.

Pulsed wave Doppler

With continuous wave Doppler, the instruments cannot discriminate depth. In contrast, a pulsed wave (PW) Doppler uses only one piezoelectric crystal (or a series of crystals working as one). The pulsed PW Doppler has the ability to discriminate Doppler signals from different depths. This happens because a pulsed wave Doppler crystal transmits intermittently, stopping to 'listen' for returning echoes between transmit cycles. The time it takes to listen to the returning echo is dependent on the depth of the vessel. Knowing the propagation speed of the US and the time it takes to listen to the returning echo, the depth of the vessel can be determined. Consequently, placement of a 'sample volume' along the axis along which the ultrasound is being emitted and received, allows for localization. This 'sample volume' is not only steerable along the axis, but its size can be varied, allowing for listening at a narrow point of flow (in a stenotic area for instance), or across the entire width of a vessel. In using pulsed Doppler, a key variable is the pulse repetition frequency (PRF), which is the number of pulse echo cycles that occur in one second, i.e. the number of times the crystal emits or listens for return information. PRF can range from several hundred to many thousands of times per second. PRF is described in hertz and 1000 pulse-echos in 1 second is 1000 Hz. One reason why PRF is important is the

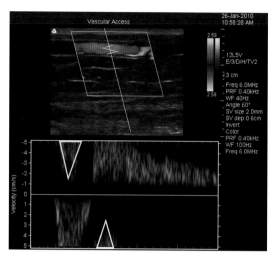

Figure 1.8 Aliasing venous Doppler signal. The yellow outline adds emphasis to show the portion of the wave form which has been 'moved' to wrap around on the other side of the baseline.

Nyquist limit, which is when the Doppler frequency shift exceeds one half of the PRF. At this limit, the waveform displayed begins 'wrapping' as noted in Figure 1.8. Interpretation of the waveform is hindered since the top has been cut off, and is being displayed as part of the bottom of the "wrapped or folded over waveform."

TIP Adjustments to eliminate aliasing can include:
- Increase the pulse repetition frequency
- Decrease the frequency shift (increase the Doppler angle)

Doppler signal spectral analysis

Blood flow in a vessel is not uniform. Although it would be easier if it were otherwise, a wide range of laminar flow and flow disturbances, and turbulence, is present in the vasculature of the body. Blood flow is faster at the center of a vessel, and slower near the walls, especially in the arterial system. In Figure 1.9, note the slower flow near the vessel wall. This flow pattern is typical of the arterial system. Venous flow is more phasic in nature, and typically at slower speeds than the arterial system.

Other venous flow disturbances resulting from valves, tortuosity, obstruction, and changes in diameter are common. The analysis of blood flow based on

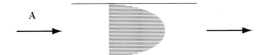

Figure 1.9 Laminar flow.

Doppler signals is now decades old. Complicated mathematical calculations using Fast Fourier transformation (FFT) processors interpret the widerange of velocities of the moving blood cells in a vessel to allow for the depiction of a spectral waveform for which standards for interpretation have developed. One such interpretation has to do with turbulent versus more laminar flow as seen mainly in arterial flow patterns. In a clear signal with a good spectral outline most of the velocities are similar, with a 'window' below the tracing line (Figure 1.10a). Whereas in a spectral image that appears 'filled in', there are more turbulent flow patterns (Figure 1.10b). It should be emphasized that these characteristics – i.e. spectral windowing – are found with arterial imaging. These concepts are not so important, or found with, venous studies. This information is presented as a basis for understanding turbulent flow. Translation of this to venous interpretation and understanding is left to the reader.

Color Duplex imaging

Spectral analysis is Doppler information converted into a waveform. Color flow imaging is a method in which a Doppler signal is presented in a different format. The waveform that we have seen previously has a positive and negative portion which is normally displayed above or below the base line, again see Figure 1.10a. In simple terms, with color flow, flow above the baseline is 'colorized' one color (perhaps blue), and flow below the baseline is colorized another color (perhaps red). This color can be superimposed on B-mode image to display the 'motion' of the blood flow in the vessel being interrogated (Figure 1.11).

With color Doppler, many (hundreds) pulsed wave Doppler signals are simultaneously interpreted. There are vast calculations and data processing which takes place in order to produce the color ultrasound image on the monitor. One aspect of this process assigns different colors to the Doppler shifts (representing the blood flow). This is known as color

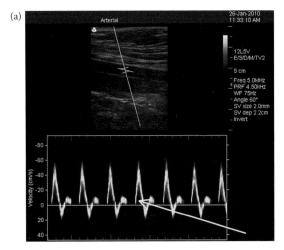

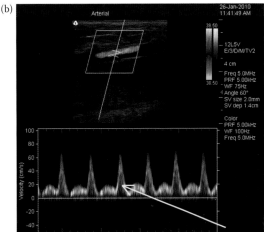

Figure 1.10 (a) Spectral windowing; (b) turbulent flow. Note adjusted Doppler angle.

encoding and directionality. In color Doppler, the color coding relates to flow towards or away from the Doppler beam. The information is assigned a color (instead of creating a waveform) and displayed as flow towards or away from the ultrasound probe, and used to 'paint' or fill in the flow within the vessel. This produces the characteristic color-filled vessel against the gray B-mode anatomic display.

The left side of Figure 1.12 shows the slanted "color box" and outlines the multiple 'listening' sites for the Doppler. Color is assigned to each site based on the movement it detects, in this case red to represent venous flow in the vein. No color is 'assigned' outside the vessel and therefore the gray image allows us to see the tissue surrounding the vein.

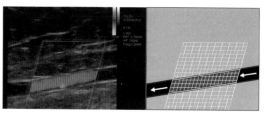

Figure 1.11 The "red" color is painted on the image where a Doppler shift occurs – i.e. inside the vessel. There is no Doppler shift outside the vessel, and therefore the surrounding tissue remains gray scale.

On the right side of Figure 1.12, the artist's grid shows the many small packets (Doppler listening areas) of information that are gathered along the 'scan lines' which are emitted from the transducer. Only in those packets where motion, and thus a Doppler shift, occurs will motion be interpreted and assigned a color. Since the blood flow is moving, the packets of information from within the vessel walls will be assigned a color, and thus we get filling in of the vessel which is interpreted as blood flow. In the absence of motion, there is no color assigned. This is why there is no color outside the vein, and if there is no flow within the vein we would see the black color of an empty lumen.

Another way of understanding the color assignment would be to colorize the spectral waveform as noted in the following figures. Forward flow is colored blue (normal) and reversed flow is red (reflux) (Figure 1.13a,b).

The blue color is related to the forward flow produced during augmentation, and the red color represents the reflux measured following release of the distal compression. If, as in Figure 1.13a, we have a normal augmentation with a short blip of flow related to valve closure, one can appreciate the larger blue triangle representing the augmentation, compared to the short area of red (reflux).

In Figure 1.13b, we see pathology. That is where the blue "normal area" is small, and the red reflux below the line, is long. In this way, we can see how a

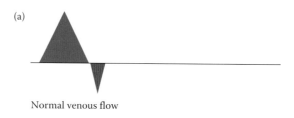

Figure 1.12 A duplex image, with to the right, an artist's representation of color sample packets in the Doppler box.

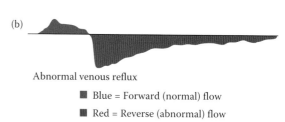

(a)

Normal venous flow

(b)

Abnormal venous reflux

■ Blue = Forward (normal) flow
■ Red = Reverse (abnormal) flow

Figure 1.13 (a,b) Color depictions of directional spectral curves.

prolonged red filling of the vein represents the longer reflux curve.

There are some newer developments in duplex technology that look at different flow patterns and characteristics. These have undetermined application to typical venous diagnosis, but are included here as an introduction. Figures 1.14–1.20 are a series of ultrasound images that are provided to additionally illustrate features and elements of duplex ultrasound and color flow dynamics.

B-mode ultrasound scanning is used to analyze the anatomy of the veins and of the surrounding tissues. Special attention is paid to the aspects of the wall and the lumen of the vein (Figure 1.14).

Pulsed wave Doppler allows measuring precisely the flux velocity. This information is displayed with a waveform and direction of blood flow is displayed above and below the base line (Figure 1.15).

Color Doppler provides real ultrasonic angiography. It allows the analysis of the direction of the flow, a qualitative analysis of the distribution of the flow velocities in the lumen of the vein and the detection of flow turbulences (Figure 1.16).

Duplex ultrasound has developed other functions or modalities which can provide additional, helpful information.

Power Doppler does not analyze the flux velocity, but only the intensity of the color Doppler signal, and eventually the direction of the flux in case of bi-directional power Doppler. This modality increases the sensitivity for detection and representation of low velocity flux (Figure 1.17).

In harmonic imaging mode, only the second harmonic of the recurrent ultrasound beam is analyzed by the ultrasound system. This modality increases

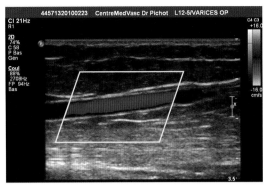

Figure 1.16 Color Doppler imaging of a normal great saphenous vein at mid-thigh demonstrating a normal antegrade flux. The color box is angulated in the flux direction in order to increase the sensitivity.

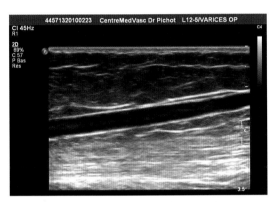

Figure 1.14 Longitudinal view of a normal great saphenous vein at mid-thigh.

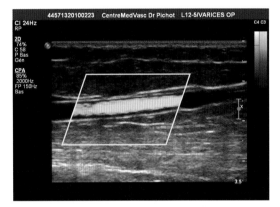

Figure 1.17 Power Doppler imaging of a normal great saphenous vein at mid-thigh. No information about the direction of the flux can be obtained, but the filling of the lumen is perfect.

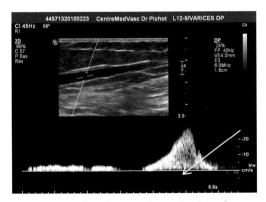

Figure 1.15 Duplex ultrasound examination of a normal great saphenous vein (GSV) at mid-thigh in the same patient. The sample volume is positioned across the whole lumen of the vein with an angle inferior to 60°. At rest, the velocity of the spontaneous flow in the GSV is nil or very low (below 5 cm/sec). It increases dramatically during the compression of the calf where indicated by the yellow arrow.

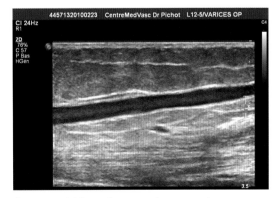

Figure 1.18 View of a normal great saphenous vein (GSV) at mid-thigh in harmonic imaging mode providing a high contrast between the vein lumen, the vein walls, and the surrounding tissues. In this case, the GSV flux is directly visible. A valve leaflet can be seen on the posterior vein wall.

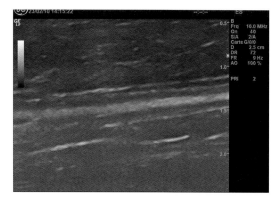

Figure 1.19 B-flow imaging of a normal great saphenous vein at mid-thigh. The flux of the vein, better analyzed on a video sequence, appears in brighter white, without clear visualization of the surrounding tissues.

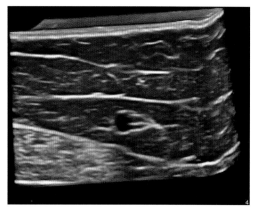

Figure 1.20 Three-dimensional imaging of a normal great saphenous vein (GSV) and surrounding tissues at mid-thigh. This B-mode reconstruction offers a transversal view of the GSV into its compartment.

the contrast and usually allows better imaging of the course of the deep or perforating veins and of venous valves in venous application (Figure 1.18).

Flux imaging

Available in several ultrasound systems, this modality (b-flow or e-flow) uses phase shift technology to obtain direct visualization of the blood flow. By focusing on flux imaging, direct tissue imaging, including the vein walls is poor. This technique allows a direct and precise analysis of the vein flux

in complex venous areas, such as vein confluences or valve implantations (Figure 1.19).

Volume ultrasound signal acquisition, required for three-dimensional imaging, can be obtained directly using a matrix probe, or from the scanning of the interest area with a linear probe in transverse view.

Three-dimensional scanning allows B mode and in some cases color or power flow reconstruction. Note to the left side of Figure 1.20, which shows the "depth" of the slice produced by 3D ultrasound. Using this technology one can "scroll" through a series of slices similar to a CT image slices.

In summary, although duplex is typically thought of as providing two 'modes' of information, color flow and the other technologies introduced briefly here provide more information. The application of these technologies has yet to be fully understood as it pertains to venous diagnosis.

REFERENCES

1. Zweibel W. *Introduction to vascular ultrasonography*, 3rd edn. Philadelphia, PA: WB Saunders, 1992: 20–2.
2. Thrush A, Hartshorne T. *Peripheral vascular ultrasound; how, why and when.* Edinburgh: Churchill Livingstone, 1999: 5–7.
3. Polak J. *Peripheral vascular sonography. A practical guide.* Philadelphia, PA: Lippincott Williams & Wilkins, 2000: 12.
4. Daigle R. *Techniques in noninvasive vascular diagnosis. An encyclopedia of vascular testing.* Littleton, CO: Summer Publishing, 2002: 1.
5. Weiss R, Feied C, Weiss M. *Vein diagnosis and treatment: a comprehensive approach.* New York: McGraw-Hill, 2001.
6. Goldman M, Bergan J, Guex JJ. *Sclerotherapy: treatment of varicose and telangiectatic leg veins,* 4th edn. Philadelphia, PA: Mosby-Elsevier, 2007.
7. Cornu-Thenard A, DeCottreau H, Weiss RA. Sclerotherapy: continuous wave Doppler-guided injections. *Dermatologic Surgery* 1995; **21**: 867–70.
8. Goldman M, Weiss R, Bergan J. *Varicose veins and telangiectasias; diagnosis and treatment,* 2nd edn. St Louis, MO: Quality Medical Publishing, 1999.

2

Venous anatomy

Any discussion on venous anatomy has to begin with a history of man's understanding of its form and function. In the second century, Galen related clear insights about venous disease and described interventions for varicose veins and venous ulcers. Although insights were noted, Galen's physiology theory spoke of 'natural spirits', and that blood was created in the liver and somehow was attracted to the extremities.[1]

Venous valves were first described in detail by Fabricius in Padua, Italy in 1579. However, it was not until the seventeenth century that a true understanding of venous flow was realized. Almost 400 years ago, in 1628, William Harvey who was studying with Fabricius in Padua, first explained one-way circulation of blood in the body. Harvey, in his treatise, *du Mortu Cordis*, described the contraction of the heart and the role of the veins in returning blood to the heart. Harvey also described the need for valves in the venous system to maintain the unidirectional aspects of blood flow. Given what Harvey taught us and the 400 years of science since, our understanding of the function and variability of the venous system continues to expand. Our understanding of venous anatomy evolved significantly almost 30 years ago with the advent of duplex ultrasound. Steve Talbot introduced B-mode imaging in 1982, focused primarily on the deep system. In the early 1990s, phlebologists began with earnest investigation of the superficial system. In 2004, renowned phlebologist Hugo Partsch said, 'duplex ultrasound is the most significant contribution to the field of phlebology in the past ten years.' Current thinking is that the venous system is actually more complex than the arterial system.[2]

Consensus on nomenclature of anatomic terms

Duplex ultrasound has especially influenced our understanding of the anatomy of the superficial and deep venous systems of the lower extremities. In 2001, an International Interdisciplinary Committee met to update and refine the *Terminologia Anatomica* concerning the lower limb veins.[3] In 2005, a follow-up article with extensions, refinements, and clinical applications was published,[4] setting the standards which are commonly employed in the international literature today. Some of the most notable revisions are encapsulated in Table 2.1.

Most notable are the elimination of the term 'superficial femoral vein' which is actually part of the deep system, and elimination of the abbreviation of LSV and terms long or lesser saphenous vein as misleading and confusing, replaced by great saphenous vein (GSV) and small saphenous vein (SSV). Another significant delineation includes the concept of the muscular fascia as a boundary between the deep and superficial compartments, and the subdivision of the superficial compartment.[5-7] A basic depiction of the saphenous compartment is noted below in Figure 2.1.

The superficial compartment now includes the 'saphenous subcompartment', described as 'duplication of the superficial fascia around the saphenous vein' and therefore always contains named saphenous vessels, and the 'true superficial compartment' which contains the epifascial tributaries. The epifascial tributaries are typically responsible for the visible varicose veins noted on clinical examination. A few eponyms, such as 'Giacomini vein', 'Cockett's perforator', and the term 'posterior arch vein' are still used worldwide in the literature,

Table 2.1 New nomenclature of key veins.

New	Old
Femoral vein	Superficial femoral vein – eliminated
Great saphenous vein	Long saphenous vein – eliminated
Inguinal confluence	Saphenofemoral junction – still used
Posterior accessory of the great saphenous vein	Posterior arch vein or vein of Leonardo
Small saphenous vein	Lesser saphenous vein – eliminated
Thigh extension of the small saphenous vein	Giacomini vein – still used
Posterior tibial perforating veins	Cockett's vein – being used less and less

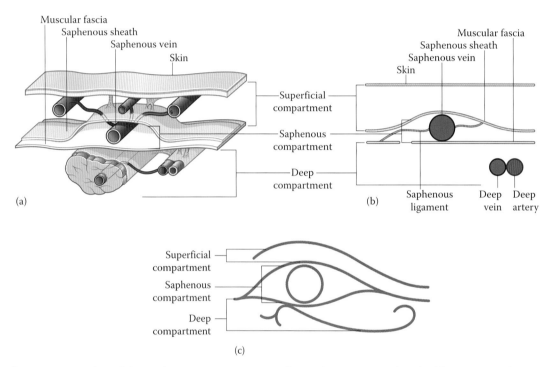

Figure 2.1 Depiction of the saphenous compartment and Egyptian eye. Reproduced with permission from Ref.10.

however most perforating veins are identified using anatomic location descriptors. Agreements on general terminology will be discussed, and specifics regarding the deep, superficial, and perforating vein systems will occur in their respective sections below.

General anatomic terms

The term **peripheral** is best used for the segment of the vein that is away from the heart, **central,** the segment of the vein towards the heart. With

regard to a duplicated vein, this term is reserved for only when the two veins display the same path, topography, and relationships (like the tibial veins). If a vein is parallel but in a different compartment or plane, it cannot be considered double, but only functionally duplicated as in the case of the femoral vein and an axial transformation of the deep femoral vein. With regard to clinical practice, duplex ultrasound helps us understand terms relating to the diameter of veins in the lower limbs. **Aplasia** refers to the absence of a vein or segment of vein. **Hypoplasia** refers to a vein diameter <50 percent of normal. Atrophy is reserved to describe a decrease in size or wasting away of a normally developed vein or vein segment – in conjunction with a degenerative process. **Dysplasia** refers to a developmental abnormality of a vein or group of veins in which size, structure, and connections are different, i.e. a venous malformation. A **venous aneurysm** is a focal dilation of a vein segment with diameter increase of >50 percent, whereas **venomegalia** is a diffuse dilation of one or more veins to >50 percent of their normal diameters.[8] Additionally, as opposed to the arterial system which bifurcates or trifurcates as one moves distal when describing its anatomy, the venous system is best understood in accordance with direction of flow, and therefore distal veins join or 'form a union' with other vessels as we move central in our descriptions (N Labropoulos, personal communication).

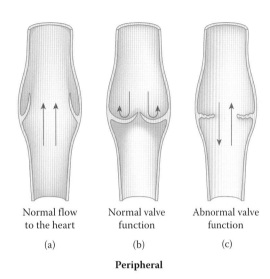

Normal flow to the heart (a)   Normal valve function (b)   Abnormal valve function (c)

Peripheral

Figure 2.2 Vein valves.

Vein valves

Normal venous valves are unidirectional and maintain blood flow towards the heart, with flow typically up and in, or from peripheral to central. Non-functioning valves or valvular dysfunction allows for reflux or retrograde flow. Most venous valves are bicuspid in nature. A vein is typically slightly dilated at a valve often described as a sinus in which we find the valve cusp or leaflets (Figure 2.2).

Duplex ultrasound allows us to understand the function of the valves and their effect on blood flow. In 2003, using ultrafast image capture (B-flow imaging), Lurie et al.[9] demonstrated and clearly described the cyclical flow events including flow separation and reattachment, and vortical flow in the sinus pocket that occur in the vein valves with the flow of blood. There are also varying flow rates in different sections of the valve structure as noted in Figure 2.3.

In summary, the valve cycle, which represents the time between two consecutive valve closures, has four distinct phases. These four phases are described in Table 2.2.

Another interesting but practical fact is that, in general, the number of valves increases the more distal in a vein one investigates. This is believed to be related to the forces of hydrostatic pressure, which increase in the periphery. When closed, the valves interrupt or segment the column of blood, compartmentalizing or fractionating the hydrostatic pressure in smaller segments (Figure 2.4).

This is intuitively confirmed the lower in the leg as one looks distally, the greater the frequency of valves is observed. Two types of valves, parietal and ostial are described. A parietal valve is located along the course of a vein in a valve sinus. For example, the calf veins have valves about every 2 cm.[1] In contrast, an ostial valve is typically found just distal to a confluence or point of union with a major tributary, such as the valve that is found in the femoral vein just distal to its union with the deep femoral vein. In the popliteal vein, there are typically two valves. In most cases, there is a valve in the great saphenous vein at its junction with the femoral vein (ostial).[10] Today, the saphenofemoral junction (SFJ) is considered to be the 'area' involving the proximal great saphenous vein that includes both the terminal and preterminal valves. Generally, the GSV has three major and up to ten minor valves, and SSV has one major valve with approximately six minor valves.[11] The veins of the foot do not have valves, which is unique.

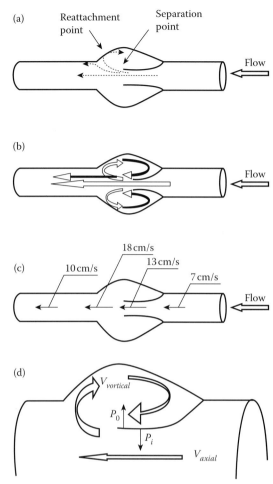

Figure 2.3 Valvular flow as described by Lurie et al.[9] (a) Flow pattern during the equilibrium phase. Flow separation at the leading edge of the cusp and reattachments at the wall of the sinus, with reflection into the sinus pocket. Flow separation is a phenomenon of flow detaching from the vessel wall and forming region of 'dead water' in which unsteady motion occurs. (b) Flow pattern during equilibrium phase. Vortex forms in sinus pocket. (c) Changes in axial velocity of flow while passing valve. Superficial femoral vein, supine position. (d) Forces acting on value leaflet. P_i, pressure applied to mural surface of valve leaflet generated by cortical flow in valve pocket, with velocity $V_{vortical}$; P_0, pressure applied to luminal surface of leaflet, generated by axial flow between leaflets, with velocity V_{axial} Reproduced from Ref.9.

Muscle pumps in the leg

Basic understanding of the leg acknowledges the presence of the calf muscle pump, sometimes called the 'peripheral heart'. Through contraction of the muscles of the calf, the veins of the lower leg are squeezed, and in keeping with the one-way valves, blood is propelled upward with muscular systole, the valves closing to prevent reflux during diastole. In contrast to arterial flow which is pulsatile, venous flow is more jerky or rachet-like, moving up in a segmented fashion between ascending valves in the deep system (Figure 2.5).

The calf pump is not the only venous pump in the leg, but it is the most described and discussed. Other pumps in the leg and the sequential systolic–diastolic phases of filling and emptying have been described. The interrelation of the foot and calf pumps is as described in Figure 2.5. More fully, the foot pump uses Lejar's plexus to empty the venous plexus of the foot. This pump is very useful in duplex imaging of the distal leg. Compression across the instep exsanguinates Lejar's plexus, emptying the foot and providing a wave of blood flow up in the deep and saphenous systems. Other pumps in the leg include the popliteal pump, the femoral vein pump, and hamstring pumps. These use the popliteus, sartorius and quadriceps, and hamstring muscles to respectively compress the popliteal, the femoral, and deep femoral veins, respectively. In unison, all of these pumps propel venous blood upwards against the forces of gravity, using the opening and closing of valves to interrupt the hydrostatic column to achieve their goal.

Deep venous system

The deep venous network is a low pressure, high volume system which is responsible for about 90 percent of the venous blood flow in the lower extremities. Deep veins are usually thinner walled veins as compared to the superficial veins, but supported by the muscles and/or the deep fascia. This forms a rigid compartment which is useful as the muscles contract in a relatively closed, inelastic space. This places pressure on the veins and 'pumps' venous blood upwards in the leg.

Table 2.2 The four phases of the valve cycle.

Opening phase	Lasting 0.27 s, in which the cusps move from the closed position towards the vein wall
Equilibrium phase	Lasting 0.65 s, in which the valves are no longer opening, but remain suspended open undergoing oscillation or fluttering in the blood flow
Closing phase	Lasting 0.41 s, in which the valves move synchronously towards the center of the vein
Closed phase	Lasting 0.45 s, in which the valve remains closed

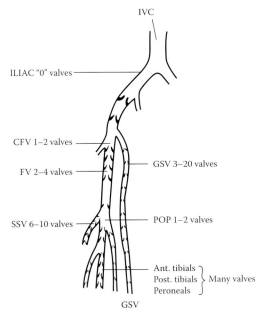

Figure 2.4 The increasing prevalence of valves in the periphery.

The deep veins of the lower extremity lie below the muscular fascia in what is referred to as the deep compartment. Although CHIVA (cure conservatrice et hemodynamique de l'insuffisance veineuse en ambulatoire) is a treatment strategy, its compartment concepts are useful. With regard to hemodynamics, the deep compartment is also referred to as the 'N1 compartment'. All deep veins are accompanied by a corresponding artery, and in the calf, are at least paired. The primary function of the deep venous system is to provide venous return to the right side of the heart. It has a large blood volume capacity (approximately three times as much as the adjacent arteries), low pressure, and compliance.[12] The pressure, volume, and flow of blood in the venous system has a tremendous impact on the shape of the vein wall. Large changes in volume (or flow) can take place with little change in pressure – which confirms the large capacitance of the venous system. Interestingly, as the veins approach a more circular distended

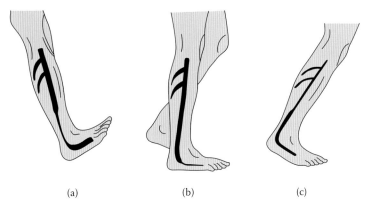

Figure 2.5 The calf and foot pump work interdependently with ambulation to propel blood upwards in the leg.

shape, a more significant pressure/volume ratio develops. This is more easily understood looking at Figure 2.6, in which volume changes versus shape of the vein are noted. This concept was originally studied in regard to flow through a collapsible tube.

As noted earlier, the consensus on nomenclature for venous anatomy was adjusted, and later refined (2005) resulting in Table 2.3, for the deep veins of the lower extremity.

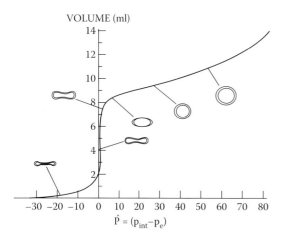

Figure 2.6 The volume–shape relationship of a vein, as related to pressure (x-axis).

Table 2.3 Nomenclature of the deep veins.

Common femoral vein
Femoral vein
Deep femoral veins
Deep femoral communicating veins
Medial circumflex femoral vein
Lateral circumflex femoral vein
Sciatic vein
Popliteal vein
Genicular venous plexus
Sural veins
Soleal veins
Gastrocmenius veins
Intergemellar vein
Anterior tibial veins
Posterior tibial veins
Peroneal veins (fibular veins)

The deep veins of the lower extremity can be divided into three parts: the leg (or calf), the thigh, and the pelvis (or suprainguinal veins). The leg includes the anterior tibial, posterior tibial, and peroneal veins, as well as the gastrocnemius and soleal veins. The thigh includes the popliteal vein, femoral vein, deep femoral vein or profunda femoris, and the common femoral vein. The pelvis includes the external iliac and common iliac veins.[13, 14] Recently, there has been much more interest in the suprainguinal veins. Advancing treatment options such as angioplasty, iliac stenting, and the application of computed tomography (CT), magnetic resonance venography (MRV), and other imaging modalities, including intravascular ultrasound (IVUS) are pushing our understanding of these areas further.

Deep veins of the leg (calf)

The anterior tibial veins drain the dorsum of the foot and course from the ankle up the anterior compartment of the leg, lateral to the tibia, and close to the interosseous membrane which connects the tibia and fibula. Near the junction of these two bones at the knee, the vessels penetrate the interosseous membrane entering the posterior compartment of the leg. Of note, isolated deep vein thrombosis (DVT) of the anterior tibial veins is very infrequent less than 2% (N Labropolous, personal communication).

The posterior tibial veins drain the medial aspect of the foot and travel upward posteromedially beneath the medial edge of the tibia. The two posterior tibial veins unite to form the common tibial trunk. The tibial veins are densely packed with valves, whereas the popliteal vein only has one or two valves, the femoral vein has between three and five valves, and the major perforating veins have between one and three valves.[14]

The peroneal veins drain the lateral aspect of the foot and travel upward posteriorly through the calf. The two peroneal veins unite to form the common peroneal trunk.

The soleal veins are the veins of the soleus muscle. They drain into either the posterior tibial or peroneal system and are a site for possibly isolated and often symptomatic venous thrombosis.

The gastrocnemius veins are divided into medial gastrocnemius vein, lateral gastrocnemius vein, and intergemellar vein (the vein ascending between the two heads of the gastrocnemius, just below the SSV). They drain into either the popliteal vein or posterior tibial system. Medial gastrocnemius veins are a site for often isolated and symptomatic venous thrombosis with, in some cases, the possibility of extension into the popliteal vein (Figure 2.7).

Deep veins of the thigh

The popliteal vein is duplicated in about 40 percent of the population,[15] and this duplication can be missed by duplex is formed by the union of the anterior and posterior tibial veins and the peroneal veins. It travels upward behind the knee and then passes anteromedially in the distal thigh through the adductor canal. The popliteal vein lies immediately posterior to the popliteal artery.

The popliteal vein becomes the femoral vein (formerly known as the superficial femoral vein) once it passes through the adductor canal. It is the largest and longest deep vein of the lower extremity. The femoral vein is bifid in approximately 25 percent of individuals.[16] Interestingly enough, although duplication may be thought to be more prone to insufficiency, actually thrombosis of the non-dominant duplicated vein is found more often. Furthermore, venous duplications may be a source of diagnostic errors as thrombus in the duplicated vein may be overlooked, and special attention needs to be paid when a vein is smaller than the expected diameter or its location atypical.[17] Sonographically from the anteromedial thigh, the femoral vein lies deep to the adjacent femoral artery.

The deep femoral vein is a short vein with its origin in the terminal muscle tributaries within the deep muscles of the lateral thigh. It is this vein which through compensatory adjustments takes up flow and becomes the outflow vein in some cases of popliteal and/or femoral vein thrombosis, or even in situations of femoral vein ligation, either planned or traumatic.

The common femoral vein is formed by the union of the femoral vein and deep femoral vein. It travels upward and becomes the external iliac vein at the inguinal ligament.

Deep veins of the pelvis

The common femoral vein becomes the external iliac vein after crossing the inguinal ligament, and dives posteriorly into the pelvis. The external iliac vein joins the internal iliac vein forming the common iliac vein.[16]

The common iliac vein is formed by the joining of the external iliac and internal iliac veins at approximately the level of the sacroiliac joints. The external iliac vein drains the lower extremity and the internal iliac vein drains the pelvis and gluteal regions.

The superficial system

Much of our understanding of the saphenous and superficial venous system is a result of the use of duplex ultrasound during the past two decades. Historically, the superficial system was anything located above the deep muscular fascia. Ultrasound, however, has allowed us to see the saphenous sheath, which forms the Egyptian eye, resulting in a duplication of the superficial fascia around the saphenous vein (Figure 2.8).[7]

Following identification of the saphenous sheath and the resulting subdivision of the superficial space, the superficial venous system is now best described based on these two subcompartments. There are true saphenous veins, which lie within

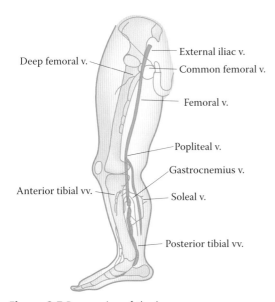

Deep femoral v.
External iliac v.
Common femoral v.
Femoral v.
Popliteal v.
Gastrocnemius v.
Anterior tibial vv.
Soleal v.
Posterior tibial vv.

Figure 2.7 Deep veins of the leg.

(a)

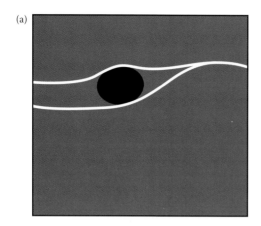

(b)

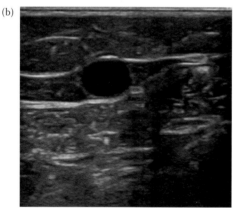

Figure 2.8 (a) Saphenous compartment; (b) corresponding duplex image.

the saphenous compartments, and superficial or epifascial tributaries which lie beneath the skin yet above this saphenous fascia. These epifascial tributaries are typically responsible for the visible varicose veins noted on clinical examination. Also, the so-called saphenous 'eye' is a key ultrasonic marker for identification of the saphenous veins. In terms of hemodynamics,[18] the saphenous compartment is known as the N2 compartment, and the epifascial space as the N3 compartment. The deep compartment is 'N1' and the direction of normal flow should be ultimately towards the N1 compartment. Figure 2.1b shows a more detailed representation of the saphenous compartment as currently understood. Note that the saphenous 'N2' compartment shows the saphenous ligament. Also noted is the saphenous nerve. In depictions that show the nerve, a common thought is the image represents the segment of the saphenous compartment in the proximal calf, as the saphenous vein is in close proximity to the saphenous vein at this level. However, if the diagram does not show a nerve, the segment is thought to be from the thigh, where the saphenous nerve typically lies in the deep compartment and slightly posterior to the saphenous vein (Figure 2.9).

As noted in other sections, the nomenclature refinements in 2005 have greatly helped academic communications, especially internationally. Table 2.4 indicates the major veins of the superficial venous system.

The great saphenous vein

The GSV begins in the foot, as a continuation of the dorsal arch vein, running from the medial ankle to the groin (Figure 2.10). More specifically, the GSV travels along the medial malleolus, up the medial calf along the tibia. At this point, it is more anterior, only moving more posterior as it nears the knee. It passes along the medial condyles of the tibia and femur slightly more posterior, and continues to ascend along the posterior portion of the thigh to the upper portion of the thigh where

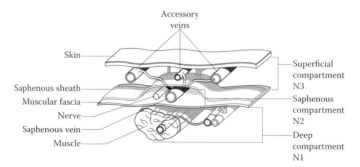

Figure 2.9 Saphenous compartment.

Table 2.4 Nomenclature of the superficial veins.

Great saphenous vein (GSV)		
Saphenofemoral junction	Terminal valve	
	Preterminal valve	
External pudendal vein		
Superficial circumflex iliac vein		
Superficial epigastric vein		
Anterior accessory of the GSV		
Posterior accessory of the GSV		
Superficial accessory of the GSV		
Small saphenous vein		
Saphenopopliteal junction	Terminal valve	
	Preterminal valve	
Cranial extension of the small saphenous vein (SSV)		
Superficial accessory of the SSV		
Anterior thigh circumflex vein		
Posterior thigh circumflex vein		
Intersaphenous veins		
Lateral venous system		
Dorsal venous network of the foot		
Dorsal venous arch of the foot		
Lateral marginal vein		
Dorsal marginal vein		

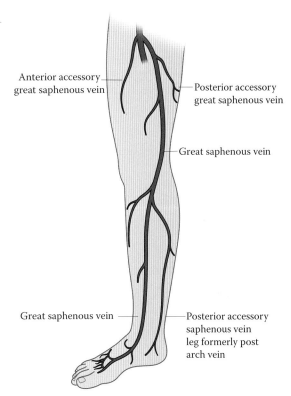

Figure 2.10 The great saphenous vein.

it turns anteriorly, descending towards the femoral vein through the fossa ovalis. At this point, it forms the saphenofemoral junction, which although fairly consistent in location, has a tremendous variability with regard to actual anatomy. Historically in the European communities, this area has also been called the 'crosse.' The term **saphenofemoral junction** is anatomically correct, not misleading and clinically appropriate, and therefore has been included in the nomenclature revisions. The saphenofemoral junction is a critical area in terms of understanding flow patterns, treatment approaches, and historical failures. This area will be discussed more fully below. It should also be noted there is segmented agenesis of the GSV in up to 16 percent of limbs.[15] This is present most often along the knee (as noted in figure 5.33).

The saphenous arch

The anatomic extent of the saphenous junction has been recently extended. The hemodynamics of the superior branches and additional understanding with recent investigations into flow patterns facilitated a need for a more refined definition of this important anatomic area. Currently, the saphenous junction, also known as the 'saphenous arch' includes the area between the terminal and preterminal valves. By definition, this also includes any of the superior branches and tributaries in this region. Figure 2.11 shows this anatomy more clearly.[10]

Also significant in this region is the anatomic variation of the saphenous arch. The superior tributaries of the arch, sometimes called the proximal tributaries are extremely variable in their presentation. These veins act as drainage for the pudendal area, lateral hip, and groin areas. There are three fairly constant SFJ tributaries, the superficial external pudendal vein, the superficial circumflex iliac vein, and superficial inferior epigastric vein. This last one, the superficial inferior epigastric vein, has

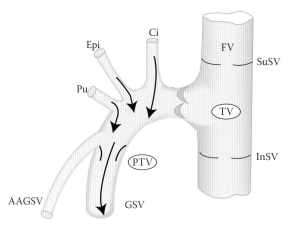

Figure 2.11 The saphenous arch. Intervalvular segment of GSV termination with tributaries: case of a preterminal reflux of the GSV trunk. AAGSV, anterior accessory saphenous vein; Ci, superficial circumflex iliac vein; Epi, superficial epigastric vein; FV, femoral vein; GSV, great saphenous vein; InSV, infrasaphenic valve; PTV, preterminal valve; Pu, external pudendal; SuSV, suprasaphenic valve; TV, terminal valve.

become increasingly important with the advent of endovenous ablation procedures. The surgical dogma of ligation and division of all junctional tributaries has been reversed, in favor of leaving these veins intact such that proper drainage, reduction of congestion, and the elimination of the release of neogenic factors will reduce the formation of neovascular clusters of varices in the groin, as often noted in recurrent varicose disease. Current thinking is that leaving the superficial inferior epigastric vein intact allows for 'washing' of the saphenofemoral junction and reduces the incidence of thrombus extension into the femoral vein following endovenous thermal ablation (Figure 2.12). There have been reported cases of thrombus extension or (endovenous heat-induced thrombus) EHIT, as described by Kabnick,[19] following thermal ablation procedures from which ongoing discussion ensues.

Reflux from the saphenous arch

With regard to reflux disease in the GSV and junctional area, some relevant facts have recently been published by Pittaluga *et al.*[20] Not only did their study confirm concepts previously presented that the presence of symptoms and extent or reflux correlated with increasing age, worsening as one

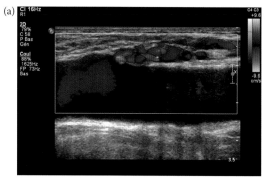

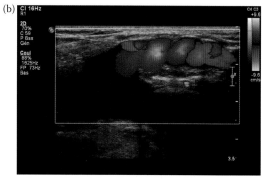

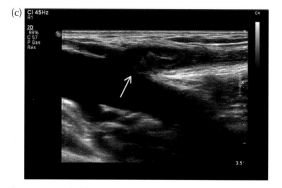

Figure 2.12 (a,b) Neovascularization as noted with the seemingly bidirectional color at the proximal GSV. Note in (a) terminal valve incompetence, (b) terminal valve and femoral vein competence. (c) EHIT (endovenous heat-induced thrombus) as described by Kabnick (19), note yellow arrow indicating proximal extension of thrombus at SFJ. Images courtesy of O Pichot MD.

Table 2.5 Localization of reflux.

	%
Great saphenous vein territory	82.7
Small saphenous vein territory	10.9
Non-saphenous territory	6.4

Reproduced from Pittaluga *et al.*[20] Another study is also presented in Table 5.3 with relatively similar figures.

ages, but several other interesting facts.[21, 22] This includes the distribution of disease noted in Table 2.5. Additionally, the distribution and prevalence of reflux of different patterns involving the absence or presence of GSV reflux with or without distal varicosities, and the incidence of the junctional or GSV vein reflux are noted in Figure 2.13.

A major distal tributary of the junctional area is the anterior accessory saphenous vein (AAGSV). This vein lies anterior to the GSV and in a saphenous compartment – sometimes a separate compartment from the GSV. Myers and Ricci described various anatomic configurations of the confluence of the GSV and AA-GSV with the femoral vein. In many cases, the AAGSV is either the origin of primary reflux or, subsequent

to initial intervention. The AAGSV, can be a source of recurrent varicose veins, and therefore is of importance in diagnosis and treatment (Figure 2.14).

The AAGSV is present in approximately 41 percent of patients. The 'alignment sign' is the anatomic marker which most easily facilitates proper identification in which the anterior accessory saphenous vein lies directly above the femoral artery and vein in the upper thigh (Figure 2.15). It should be noted that in some instances the AAGSV is larger, and thus more dominant in presentation, especially when the GSV is normal or hypoplastic.

Other distal venous tributaries of the GSV have one of two presentations. Epifascial tributary veins that run parallel to the GSV are called **accessory**

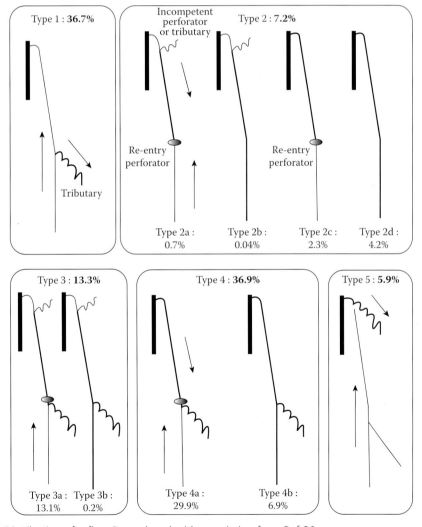

Figure 2.13 Distribution of reflux. Reproduced with permission from Ref.20.

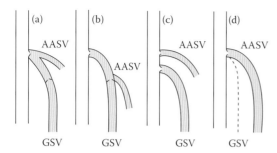

Figure 2.14 Variations in origin of the anterior accessory saphenous vein (AASV). (a) Common junction with great saphenous vein (GSV); (b) origin from GSV below saphenofemoral junction (SFJ); (c) origin from common femoral vein (CFV) above SFJ; (d) origin from SFJ as principal vein with hypoplastic or absent GSV – reproduced Ref 26.

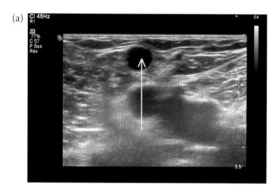

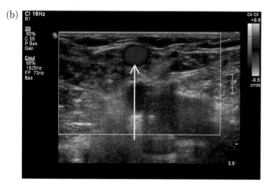

Figure 2.15 The alignment sign in gray-scale duplex, with the corresponding color duplex image. Note the alignment of the anterior accessory saphenous vein (AASV) above the deep vessels of the thigh (yellow arrow added for emphasis). Image courtesy of J Zygmunt RVT RPhS.

veins, while veins that run oblique to the saphenous compartment are called **circumflex veins**. In the upper thigh, there is the anterior thigh circumflex vein that runs oblique to the saphenous towards the lateral thigh. There is also the posterior thigh circumflex vein which courses posterior to the posterior thigh, which may be the proximal end of the intersaphenous vein, sometimes called the vein of Giacomini.

In the lower portion of the leg, the great saphenous is joined by two other tributaries: the posterior accessory saphenous vein of the leg, previously called the posterior arch vein or vein of Leonardo, and the anterior accessory saphenous vein of the leg. Clinically important, the posterior accessory saphenous vein is most often involved with the Cockett or posterior tibial perforating veins in the presentation of venous ulceration. This point needs to be stressed as it is commonly not well appreciated by novices. *In most instances, the distal great saphenous vein does not connect to the Cockett or posterior tibial perforators.* Almost universally, the posterior tibial perforators connect the posterior tibial veins and the posterior accessory saphenous vein (previously the posterior arch vein). (This is more fully illustrated below in Figure 2.21 under Perforating veins).

With regard to saphenous anatomy, and specifically for duplex imaging and endovenous ablations, the distribution of the saphenous vein in its compartment with variations will be discussed next. Typical presentation of the GSV and its tributaries falls into three distinct patterns as previously described by Ricci and Caggiati[23] as type 'I', 'h', or 'S'. In the 'I' presentation, the saphenous trunk is noted continuously throughout the entire saphenous compartment from ankle to groin with no large tributaries. This is the pattern found in approximately 50 percent of cases. The 'h' presentation is similar to the 'I' presentation, but with the addition of a large tributary of the saphenous vein, and represents about 25 percent of cases. The tributary is often larger in diameter than the saphenous trunk, and can be located anterior or posterior to the native GSV, with its origin at varying levels. Lesser prevalent is the 'S'-type presentation in which a superficial tributary becomes dominant, and the GSV is either absent or hypotrophic (Figure 2.16). It should be noted that true duplication of the GSV in the saphenous sheath, although previously reported higher, is very uncommon – currently reported to be 1–2 percent.[24, 25]

In approximately 70 percent of patients, the GSV is present from groin to ankle within the saphenous compartment. Variations in which the GSV is hypotrophic or absent in the distal thigh and proximal calf account for the remaining 30 percent. Myers'

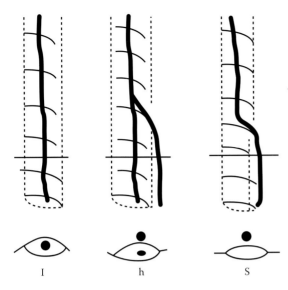

Figure 2.16 The relationship of the great saphenous vein (GSV), sheath, and major tributaries: the 'I' type, the 'h' type, and the 'S' type.

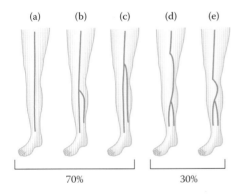

Figure 2.17 Great saphenous vein (GSV) present to the ankle: (a) no major tributaries; (b) one of two major tributaries below the knee; (c) a major tributary above the knee. GSV is present continuously at the knee: (d) absence of significant portion of GSV above and below knee; (e) absence of a short length of GSV above and below the knee. Reproduced with permission from Ref.26.

description of the typical presentations of the GSV in the distal thigh and proximal calf are described in Figure 2.17.[26]

The small saphenous vein

The SSV has its origin in the lateral marginal foot vein and continues posteriorly up the leg starting behind the lateral malleolus. This vein ascends in its own fascial compartment similar to the GSV (Figure 2.18).

The SSV fascial compartment varies in size as it ascends, being wider and most easily seen in the midcalf, but thinning significantly as it nears the popliteal fossa, making it difficult to identify. The SSV joins the deep system at the popliteal vein; however, this anatomy is quite variable, with several presentations. These presentations fall into one of three presentations: (1) The SSV joins the popliteal vein at the saphenopopliteal junction (SPJ) with a thigh extension (TE) ascending up the posterior thigh. (2) The SSV ascends up the posterior thigh as the TE with only a hypoplastic anastomotic vein connected to the popliteal vein. These first two presentations account for about 75 percent of the population. (3) Where the SSV continues up the posterior thigh as the TE without any connection to the popliteal vein, about 25 percent of the population. This thigh extension or Giacomini vein ascends the posterior thigh in its own fascial sheath (Figure 2.19).

The location of the SPJ is predominantly above the popliteal crease, however it is often variable. Myers published a summary of his findings on location of the SPJ with relation to the popliteal crease (Figure 2.20).[26]

The thigh extension or Giacomini vein was first described by Giacomini in 1873. This vein ascends the posterior thigh and, in the upper thigh, can travel medially to join the posterior circumflex saphenous vein, the true Giacomini vein. Other variants of the thigh extension include; diving to join the profunda femoris vein, or divide in many muscular, subcutaneous, or even continue as the gluteal vein(s).

A tributary of note is the so-called 'lateral small saphenous vein', which was first described by Dodd as a 'popliteal fossa perforating vein'. This vessel runs in a fascial compartment located lateral to the small saphenous vein. It runs parallel to the small saphenous and often has its own junction with the popliteal vein. Due to this parallel orientation, it can be dubbed the lateral accessory small saphenous vein. On a purely anecdotal note, the author's experience with this vein is that it can be very symptomatic and contribute significantly to lateral ankle edema when refluxing. This is probably due to its close association with the common peroneal nerve. One should also note that thickening of the distal SSV (vein wall) is a sign of chronic venous hypertension as noted by Raffetto and Khalil.[27]

(a)

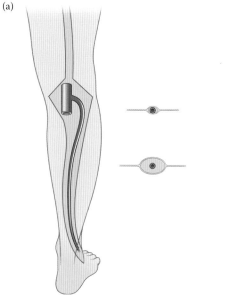

(b)

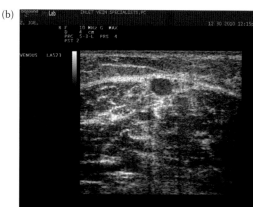

(c)

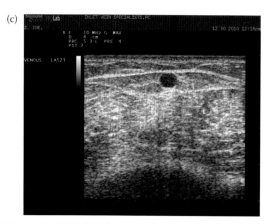

Figure 2.18 (a) Line drawing of small saphenous vein (SSV) with adjacent two duplex images (b) one high (thinner facial space fascia) and (c) one from the mid-calf with a wider fascial space.

(a)   (b)

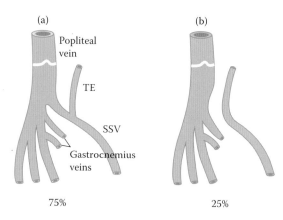

75%   25%

Figure 2.19 Small saphenous vein (SSV): variations in its termination: The thigh extension (TE) is present in 95 percent of limbs and is the continuation of the SSV. (a) The SSV may join the popliteal vein or deep veins at a higher level. (b) There may be no connection to deep veins. The SSV may be in the midline, or medial or lateral to the midline. The gastrocnemius veins may join the popliteal vein, upper SSV, or confluence at the saphenopopliteal junction (SPJ). Reproduced with permission from Ref.26.

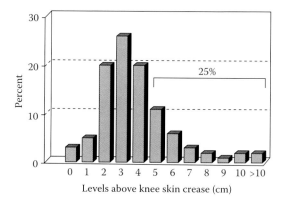

Figure 2.20 Small saphenous vein. Level of SPJ: is variable; is most often 2–4 cm above the knee crease; 25 percent are higher than this level; junction is rarely below the knee crease.

Perforating veins

Perforating veins (PV) are veins which connect the superficial and deep veins. They complete the circuit between the superficial (N2) and deep (N1) compartments as they perforate the muscular fascia. They have valves that normally prevent reflux of blood from the deep veins into the superficial system.[13] The term **communicating veins** should only

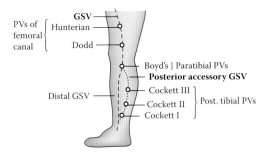

Figure 2.21 Perforating veins. The old perforating names (eponyms) and the correct anatomic names of the Pvs noted.

be used to describe veins that interconnect with other veins of the same system (or compartment). Perforating veins are numerous and very variable in arrangement, connection, and size (Figure 2.21).

In normally functioning perforating veins, valves maintain flow in one direction, from superficial to deep. Flow in the opposite direction is always abnormal. Perforators are most numerous below the knee and are of clinical importance if incompetent, permitting blood to flow from the deep to the superficial system. Perforator incompetence is always associated with superficial varicosities, as well as discoloration, thickening, and ulceration of the skin.[22, 28]

The old nomenclature used the name of the person (eponyms) who discovered the perforating veins, and this has been discouraged. The updated and refined nomenclature uses the location of the perforating vein. These can be grouped on the basis of their topography and named according to their location. The six main groups based on topography are the foot, ankle, leg (calf), knee, thigh, and gluteal perforators (see Table 2.6).

The cause of perforator insufficiency is not known and its importance is still debatable. In the presence of incompetence, perforators serve as a pressure release or equilibrium point between the two compartments. The exact location of perforators should be described by measuring their distance from a fixed anatomical point.[22] While agreeing with several other authors, Labropoulos et al.[29] reports the following facts regarding perforating veins:

- With increasing severity of chronic venous disease (CVD), the size of PVs increases.
- With increasing severity of CVD, the number of PVs increases.
- As a PV progresses from competent to incompetent, there is progression of the patient's CVD, and an increase in PV size.

Table 2.6 Updated nomenclature using the location of the perforating vein (PV).

Main groups	Perforators by location
Foot	Dorsal foot or intercapitular PV
	Medial foot, lateral foot, plantar foot PV
Ankle	Medial ankle, lateral ankle, anterior ankle PV
Leg (calf)	Medial leg: paratibial[a] (Sherman, Boyd), posterior tibial PV[b] (Cockett)
	Anterior leg,[c] lateral leg PV,[d] posterior leg PV (medial and lateral gastrocnemius, intergemellar, para-achillean PV)
Knee	Medial knee, suprapatellar, lateral knee, infrapatellar, popliteal fossa PV
Thigh	Medial thigh: PV of the femoral canal (Dodd), inguinal PV
	Anterior thigh, lateral thigh PV
	Posterior thigh: posteromedial, sciatic, posterolateral PV
Gluteal	Superior gluteal, midgluteal, lower gluteal PV

[a] Paratibial perforators connect the main trunk or tributaries of the great saphenous vein (GSV) and course close to the medial surface of the tibia (so-called Sherman perforating vein (PV)).

[b] Posterior tibial perforators ((upper, middle, and lower), formerly the Cockett PV) connect the posterior accessory GSV with the PTV.

[c] Anterior leg perforators connect the anterior tributaries of the GSV to the anterior tibial vein (ATV).

[d] Lateral leg perforators connect veins of the lateral venous plexus with the fibular veins.

- Progression of disease, measured over 25 months in this report, confirmed reflux patterns are not static.
- Correction of superficial incompetence can correct PV and possibly deep vein incompetence.

Parks also reported that after saphenous vein ablation, only 33 percent of perforators that were incompetent prior to surgery, remained incompetent following intervention. Of note in that study, this reversal of incompetence was size dependent, with all perforators over 4 mm remaining incompetent following saphenous ablation.[30] Overall, there is still much discussion and debate on perforator insufficiency, and the timing and necessity for direct treatment of PVs remains unclear. The advent of endovenous thermal ablation has further fueled this discussion.[31] More recently, the combined statement from the American Venous Forum and Society of Vascular Surgery defined a pathologic perforator which, among other things, needs to be located underneath healed or active ulceration.[32] There certainly can be a place for thermal ablation of incompetent perforators in higher risk C4–C6 patients as compared to SEPS (subfascial endoscopic perforator surgery) as noted in these guidelines.

Variations of venous anatomy

Variations of any of the preceding anatomic descriptions are common. In this next brief section, variations of the SFJ or saphenous arch configurations and venous malformations, as well as pelvic congestion will be briefly discussed.

The anatomy of the saphenous arch described previously was the classic version regarding the valves and tributaries. However, the variability of the position of the circumflex iliac, epigastric, and pudendal veins is well known.[14] Current thinking is that three factors working in conjunction are probably responsible for a vast majority of the recurrence and failure with historical surgical treatment approaches. When we see the myriad of anatomic variations, it is easy to appreciate incomplete or inaccurate surgical dissection during ligation and division prior to vein stripping. We are acquiring more and more information on frustrated abdominal wall drainage, with the advent of endovenous thermal ablation,

now that the epigastric vein is being 'left untouched' to drain and wash the stump of the SFJ. We add to that the release of angiogenic factors which occur with vessel injury – as with ligation division – and it is easy to understand why extensive neovascularization and recurrence occurs in the groin. One last factor is, of course, the advent of duplex ultrasound which allows for easy and repeatable investigation of the saphenous arch. Shown here are some variations on the veins of the saphenous arch (Figure 2.22).

With regard to venous malformations, this can be an entire field of study in and of itself. Lee *et al.*[33] recently described the variations of congenital vascular malformations, of which there are arteriovenous malformations, venous malformations, or lymphatic malformations. There are two broad categories of venous malformations: truncular and extratruncular.[34] Extratruncular venous malformations develop from embryologic remnants and are infiltrative in nature. Truncular venous malformations develop later and are typically more defined. Both malformations typically have dilated and

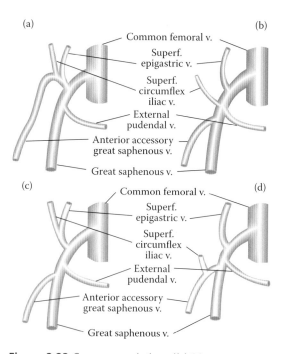

Figure 2.22 Common variations ((a) 33 percent; (b) 15 percent; (c) 15 percent; (d) 13 percent) in the anatomy of the confluence of inguinal veins (saphenofemoral junction). Reproduced with permission from Ref.14.

valveless venous channels with retrograde flow leading to pain, swelling, and varicosities. When it comes to the lower extremities, venous malformations are often affiliated with varicosities and for this reason are often misdiagnosed. The key for duplex differentiation would be the multiple or affiliated venous channels that *coexist* with pathologic superficial veins. If well diagnosed and appreciated on duplex, a more thorough work up with magnetic resonance imaging (MRI) or other imaging techniques is usually necessary to complete the analysis of the malformation before treatment.

In a similar manner, patients with pelvic congestion syndrome often present with a variant of varicosities of the upper posteromedial thigh. These varices often connect to the great saphenous vein, developing reflux along the course of the GSV. In this instance, the central or proximal source can be overlooked by the novice investigator. A good clinical history can often point to a pelvic issue in which studies, in addition to duplex, are warranted. The key fact here is that traditional duplex investigation does not routinely provide the information to ascertain this information. Varices of the upper posterior-medial thigh are particularly suggestive of pelvic origin, which spill down the posterior thigh. These are all clues for the astute phlebology sonographer. Other imaging modalities are typically needed to understand suprainguinal contributions (Figure 2.23).

Another key clue to the pelvic component is the patient's symptoms. Rosenblatt (personal communication) describes the presence of pelvic symptoms as a key factor in suggesting a proximal or central source when varices of the upper thigh are noted. These symptoms can be worsened with treatment of the distal areas, basically causing more congestion, and suggest the need for central investigation.

The new nomenclature of the anatomy of the pelvic venous system was described in 2010.[35] This article recaps the breakthrough in the understanding of these important and sometimes overlooked sources of venous reflux. Leak points in the pelvic anatomy are further described by Franceschi as the 'pelvic shunts'.[36] Pelvic shunts are the result of pelvic escape points (PEP) and are sometimes an overlooked source of varicose veins.[37] The pelvic escape points are identified and named in relation to their location (anatomic format) and their sources, i.e. the tributaries of the hypogastric veins. There are four pelvic escape points (Figure 2.24). There are two main areas of leakage as described below (P and I) and two minor points (O and G):

■ I point (IP) – or inguinal point – located at the superficial inguinal orifice and fed by the round ligament vein, and can link with veins of

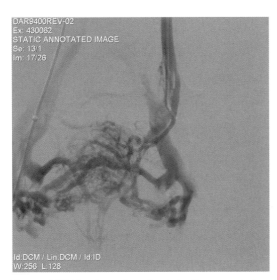

Figure 2.23 Ovarian vein reflux into the parauterine varices classic in pelvic congestion. Image courtesy of Stephen Daugherty MD RVT.

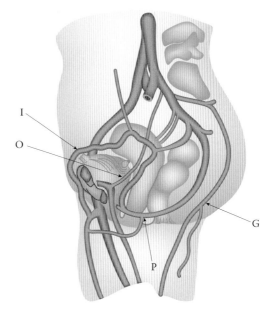

Figure 2.24 Pelvic escape points. Reproduced with permission from Ref.35. This shows the I (inguinal), O (obturator), P (perineal) and G (gluteal) leak points.

the abdominal wall and the tributaries of the saphenous arch.

- P point (PP) – or perineal point – located at the perineal membrane and fed by the pudendal vein, and can be linked to vulvar, perineal, and scrotal varices.
- O point (OP) – located in the thigh usually with the common femoral vein, having its reflux from the obturator vein. This reflux is commonly dumped into the deep system, but may also link to the saphenous arch.
- The G points are sometimes described as superior and inferior.
- SG point (SGEP) – or superior gluteal escape point – is located at the mid-portion of the buttock and typically linked to congenital varices that can involve the SSV.
- IG point (IGEP) – or inferior gluteal escape point – is located at the infragluteal fold region and can feed varices of the sciatic nerve.

The leakage points described above are clinically important in the diagnosis of reflux. There are multiple communications through venous plexuses horizontally and vertically, also connecting one side of the body with the other, so closure of one P point may not fully eradicate these refluxes. Pregnancy has a significant influence on these patterns. Any 'proximal' source could meander in a variety of pathways to connect with either the saphenous arch, axial saphenous veins, or other superficial venous anatomy. When these reflux points exist, they are often in parallel with traditional saphenous reflux patterns and may be underappreciated.

REFERENCES

1. Tretbar LL. *Venous disorders of the legs, principles and practice.* London: Springer, 1999.
2. Meissner M, Moneta G, Burnand K *et al.* The hemodynamics and diagnosis of venous disease. *Journal of Vascular Surgery* 2007; **46**: 4S–24S.
3. Caggaiti A, Bergan JJ, Gloviczki P *et al.* Nomenclature of the veins of the lower limbs: an international interdisciplinary consensus statement. *Journal of Vascular Surgery* 2002; **36**: 416–22.
4. Caggaiti A, Bergan JJ, Gloviczki P *et al.* Nomenclature of the veins of the lower limb:

extensions, refinements, and clinical application. *Journal of Vascular Surgery* 2005; **41**: 719–24.
5. Coleridge-Smith P, Labropoulos N, Partsch H *et al.* Duplex ultrasound investigation of the veins in chronic venous disease of the lower limbs – UIP Consensus Document. Part I. Basic principles. *European Journal of Vascular and Endovascular Surgery* 2006; **31**: 83–92.
6. Caggiatti A, Bergan JJ. The saphenous vein: derivation of its name and relevant anatomy. *Journal of Vascular Surgery* 2002; **35**: 172–5.
7. Caggiati A, Ricci S. The long saphenous vein compartment. *Phlebology* 1997; **12**: 107–11.
8. Zygmunt J. What's new in duplex scanning of the venous system. *Perspectives in Vascular Surgery and Endovascular Therapy* 2009; **21**: 94–104.
9. Lurie F, Kistner R, Eklof B, Kessler D. Mechanism of venous valve closure and role of the valve in circulation: a new concept. *Journal of Vascular Surgery* 2003; **38**: 955–61.
10. Uhl JF, Gillot C. Embryology and three dimensional anatomy of the superficial venous system. *Phlebology* 2007; **22**: 194–206.
11. Browse NL, Burnand KG, Irvine AT *et al. Diseases of the veins.* London: Arnold, 1999.
12. Pieri A, Gatti M, Santini M *et al.* Ultrasonographic anatomy of the deep veins of the lower extremity. *Journal of Vascular Technology* 2002; **26**: 201–11.
13. Fronek H. *The fundamentals of phlebology: venous disease for clinicians,* 2nd edn. London: Royal Society of Medicine Press, 2008.
14. Bergan J. *The vein book.* Burlington, MA: Elsevier Academic Press, 2007.
15. Malgor RD, Labroponlas N. Diagnosis and follow-up of varicose veins with duplex ultrasound: how and why? *Phlebology* 2012; **27** (suppl 1): 10–15.
16. Zwiebel WJ. *Introduction to vascular ultrasonography,* 3rd edn. Philadelphia, PA: WB Saunders, 1992.
17. Paraskevas, P, Femoral vein duplications: incidence and potential significance. *Phlebology* 2011; **26**: 52–5.
18. Francheschi C. *Theorie et pratique de la cure conservatrice et hemodynamique de l'insuffisance veineuse en ambulatiore.* Precy-sous-Thil: Editions de l'Armancon, 1988.

19. Kabnick LS. Complications of endovenous therapies: statistics and treatment. *Vascular* 2006; **14**: S31–32.
20. Pittaluga P, Chastanet S, Rea B, Barbe R. Classification of saphenous refluxes: implications for treatment. *Phlebology* 2008; **23**: 2–9.
21. Labropoulos N, Leon M, Nicolaides AN *et al.* Superficial venous insufficiency: correlation of anatomic extent of reflux with clinical symptoms and signs. *Journal of Vascular Surgery* 1994; **20**: 953–8.
22. Labropoulos N, Leon L, Kwon S *et al.* Study of venous reflux progression. *Journal of Vascular Surgery* 2005; **25**: 53–9.
23. Ricci S, Caggiati A. Does a double saphenous vein exist? *Phlebology* 1999; **14**: 59–64.
24. Cavezzi A, Labropoulos N, Partsch H *et al.* Duplex ultrasound investigation of chronic venous disease of the lower limbs – UIP Consensus Document. Part II Anatomy. *Phlebology* 2006; **21**: 168–79.
25. Labropoulous N, Kokkosis A, Spentzouris G *et al.* The distribution and significance of varicosities in the saphenous trunks. *Journal of Vascular Surgery* 2010; **51**: 96–103.
26. Myers K, Clough A. *Making sense of vascular ultrasound.* London: Arnold, 2004.
27. Raffetto JD, Khalil RA. Mechanisms of varicose vein formation: valve dysfunction and wall dilation. *Phlebology* 2008; **23**: 85–98.
28. Hannon K, Iafrati M, Mackey W. Complex lower-extremity venous disease. *Journal for Vascular Ultrasound* 2006; **30**: 167–9.
29. Labropoulos N, Tassiopoulos A, Bhatti A, Leon L. Development of reflux in the perforator veins in limbs with primary venous disease. *Journal of Vascular Surgery* 2006; **43**: 558–62.
30. Parks T, Lamka C, Nordestgaard A. Changes in perforating vein reflux after saphenous vein ablation. *Journal for Vascular Ultrasound* 2008; **32**: 141–4.
31. O'Donnell T. The role of perforators in chronic venous insufficiency. *Phlebology* 2010; **25**: 3–10.
32. Gloviczki P, Comerota AJ, Glociczki MC *et al.* The care of patients with varicose veins and associated chronic venous dieases: clinical practice guidelines of the Society for Vascular Surgery and the American Venous Forum. *Journal of Vascular Surgery* 2011; **53**: 2S–48S.
33. Lee BB, Lardeo J, Neville R. Arteriovenous malformation: how much do we know? *Phlebology* 2009; **24**: 193–200.
34. Rosenblatt M. Endovascular management of venous malformations. *Phlebology* 2007; **22**: 264–75.
35. Kachlik D, Pechacek V, Musil V, Baca V. The venous system of the pelvis: new nomenclature. *Phlebology* 2010; **25**: 162–73.
36. Franceschi C, Zamboni P. *Principles of venous hemodynamics.* New York: Nova Biomedical, 2009.
37. Liddle AD, Davies AH. Pelvic congestion syndrome: chronic pelvic pain caused by ovarian and internal iliac varices. *Phlebology* 2007; **22**: 100–4.

3

Indirect non-invasive venous testing

Non-invasive venous testing can generally be broken down into two areas: indirect tests, including plethysmography, and direct testing, which includes B-mode and duplex, which consists of spectral analysis of Doppler signals with or without color flow analysis.

Indirect tests

On a broader scale, indirect non-invasive flow studies have been slowing losing favor in the world of phlebology. They should, however, be understood, as some aspects are still applicable. There are still a few academics who stress the value of the information provided by these studies.[1, 2] With expanding interest in deep venous disease and quantifying the extent of deep disease in evaluating the risk–benefits of intervention, application of air plethysmography (APG) testing parameters may regain interest and benefit. There could currently be phlebologic research done with these plethysmographic determinations and the efforts of these academics should be applauded.

Most indirect non-invasive testing is based on plethysmographic techniques, which put simply means that they measure volume change, in this case the venous volume in the lower extremity. As an aside, these studies are coded and billed as 93965, although there is some confusion, the American Medical Association (AMA) manual on CPT (current procedural terminology) coding indicates that plethysmography codes require a separate and distinct piece of equipment (from the duplex scanner). There are four basic types of plethysmography that each work on slightly different principles. With each of these devices, venous determinations typically involve placing a measuring device on the calf (leg). With some of these techniques, there is often a cuff placed over the thigh to occlude the deep system as well. Over the course of time, with or without specific maneuvers, the lower portion of the device measures changes in volume from which interpretations are made, and measurements of different venous flow parameters can be determined: venous volume (VV), venous refilling times (VRT), maximum venous outflow (MVO), segmental venous capacitance (SVC), and the ejection fraction (EF) can also be determined.[3, 4]

Impedence plethysmography (IPG) has its basis in electronics and impedance of a current across a segment. By measuring the voltage of a microcurrent across a segment of the limb and comparing this to known standards, assumptions can be made about the current over the segment. Although blood, bone, and all subcutaneous tissue have impedance, with an assumption that only blood flow changes over time of the test duration, then the measurement of this voltage is proportional to venous volume in the limb. This can be a technically challenging device to use. With the advent of duplex ultrasound, this technique has fallen out of favor.

Strain-gauge plethysmography (SPG) is based on circumference measurements performed with strain gauges. A strain gauge is made with small mercury-filled tubes through which the device passes a microcurrent. By measuring the circumference of the calf over time, venous blood volume (again assumed to be the only variable) can be determined. Similar to the IPG, the SPG has technical challenges. Combined with the advent of direct visualization of the deep system with duplex, these challenges have also influenced their decline in use (Figure 3.1).

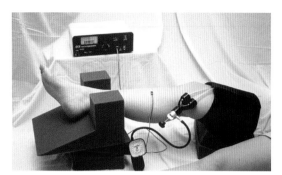

Figure 3.1 Strain-gauge plethysmography, showing patient position. Image courtsey Hokanson.

Photoplethysmography (PPG) is a technique that does not allow for the measurement of maximum venous outflow (MVO), but is still used in some vein clinics due to its ability to detect venous insufficiency. If coupled to direct current (DC), venous flow can be measured, while with the use of alternating current (AC), arterial flow can be investigated. This technique is relatively more indirect. The transducer emits light into the skin, which is scattered, absorbed, and reflected. The intensity of reflected light is diminished with higher blood content in the tissue. Typically, the transducer is placed above the medial malleolus for venous insufficiency determinations. With dorsiflexion (muscular contraction), blood leaves the calf in the venous system. During relaxation, venous refilling takes place. If venous valves are competent, venous refilling takes longer, filling through the arterial tree. However, if venous incompetence of the valves is present, venous refilling is more rapid.

Figure 3.2 shows two PPG tracings. The upper tracing shows the baseline and emptying of the calf with exercise (downward step-like deflections) and the return to baseline as the graph climbs on the right side. This upper tracing is about 10 seconds in duration which is short, indicating insufficiency. The lower tracing shows the same downward step deflections, with a slower and more gradual return taking 26 seconds. This slower return to baseline is indicative of normal venous flow. The downward deflections in both graphs, i.e. the drop from baseline indicate good venous emptying of the calf (Figure 3.2).

Table 3.1 provides information for interpretation of venous reflux based on the refilling times.

As noted above, the shape of the left side of the curve with the stepward lowering measures ejection of blood volume from the calf. If this 'ejection' does not occur well, the downward deflections are not as dramatic and this shows evidence of poor calf muscle pump function, another important hemodynamic factor. When using PPG, a determination is often performed, and if abnormal a tourniquet is placed above the knee and the test is repeated. In theory, the tourniquet compresses the great saphenous vein eliminating its contribution to reflux. If the study normalizes, this is diagnostic of great saphenous vein (GSV) reflux. If, however, the study continues to be abnormal, deep system incompetence is suggested. This is a crude assumption because with a thigh tourniquet, a small saphenous incompetence, or actually a large GSV incompetent perforator below the

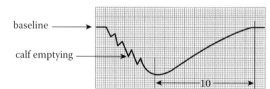

This tracing shows a short refilling time of only 10 seconds

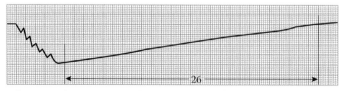

This tracing being 26 seconds long is suggestive of normal valvular function

Figure 3.2 Typical photoplethysmography (PPG) tracing.

Table 3.1 Photoplethysmography venous refilling times.

>25 seconds	Normal
20–25 seconds	Mild venous insufficiency
10–19 seconds	Moderate venous insufficiency
<10 seconds	Severe venous insufficiency

position of the tourniquet could result in a continued abnormal result, producing a false positive for deep vein incompetence. This illustrates the concept by which multiple tourniquets or multiple repeat examinations with placing the tourniquet in several different locations is espoused to facilitate differentiation of disease. With the advent of duplex, some of these misconceptions can be eliminated if using both techniques in a complementary manner. One must remember, however, that PPG is an indirect evaluation and specific anatomic variations could explain many variations in the results. Light reflective rheography (LRR) and digital photoplethysmography (D-PPG) are variations on these same principles. Typically, the LRR or D-PPG tracings appear to be inverted (mirror image) as compared to the tracing above. As already mentioned, PPG can also be used to detect arterial flow. If the PPG is coupled with AC, then arterial pulsations are able to be measured. Using AC, flow in the digits and toes can be measured for arterial insufficiency, e.g. diabetic arterial insufficiency due to calcification of the tibial arteries or Raynaud's syndrome.

Air plethysmography (APG) is another plethysmographic technique for venous flow, used primarily in academic settings. This examination, while technically difficult to perform, does provide good hemodynamic information. An improvement over the PPG technique, this method has a larger sampling area due to the design and cuff size. With APG, an air chamber (APG cuff) is placed around the calf and inflated. Another smaller air-sensing chamber is placed between the leg and this larger chamber as noted in Figure 3.3.

Over time, the APG provides several data points regarding venous flow parameters. Figure 3.4 shows the changing position of the patient (1–4), which account for some of the technical challenges with this technique. However, when done well, in addition to the data already mentioned,

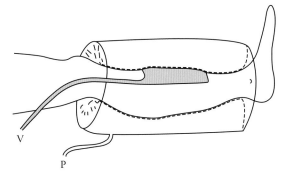

Figure 3.3 Air plethysmography cylinder encompassing the calf, showing the limb volume sensor (V) and pressure source (P).

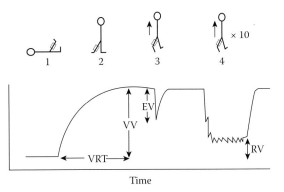

Figure 3.4 Parameter definitions and maneuvers used generically in plethysmographic studies for venous insufficiency.

the APG will also provide measurement of the ejection volume (EV) and residual volume (RV), and venous filling index (VFI). Ejection volume and ejection fraction are measures which help in the evaluation of muscle pump function. With a failed calf muscle pump, both the EV and EF are reduced, however the residual volume RV remains high. A residual volume fraction (RVF) of <35 percent is associated with normal venous subjects, whereas a RVF of >35 percent is indicative of increased venous hypertension and requires further evaluation. Venous filling index is calculated by taking 90 percent VV/ VFT90 which is the time required to achieve 90 percent of venous volume (Figure 3.4).

The calculations provide an advantage with this method in the ability to quantify reflux with VFI in a global hemodynamic manner, as opposed to duplex ultrasound which allows for interrogation of individual veins. Although APG provides this additional information, as stated above, its use is typically limited to academic or hospital settings. There are several authors who believe that a combination of duplex with APG provides further information useful to the clinician.[5] Table 3.2 below shows interpretation criteria for APG studies.[6]

A long-term study used APG to evaluate changes in venous hemodynamics after treatment of primary varicose veins. This study clearly demonstrated improvement of venous reflux and calf muscle function with primary intervention for varicose veins.[7] The study demonstrated the value of the information gathered with this important venous testing modality.

Direct testing with ultrasound

Direct testing, in contrast to indirect testing, involves the investigation of specific veins and their characteristics. Direct testing is performed using B-mode duplex ultrasound. When color flow is added, this becomes triplex ultrasound, although some purists prefer the term 'color flow duplex imaging'. Other imaging techniques with specific applications, including venography, ascending or descending, magnetic resonance imaging (MRI), and computed tomography (CT) are complementary methods and will not be discussed.

Duplex imaging includes two separate and distinct parts, B-mode gray scale imaging and spectral analysis. The B-mode is what 'paints' the picture allowing us to distinguish anatomic variations, and spectral imaging provides for the interpretation and understanding of blood flow parameters. These aspects have been discussed previously.

Direct testing with intravascular ultrasound

Intravascular ultrasound (IVUS) is a relatively new technology and is becoming more widely used. As it is more expensive than duplex, its uses are more limited. It is especially helpful in the iliac and inferior vena cava with regard to deep disease. The recent UIP (International Union of Phlebology) consensus document of deep venous treatment provided much information on our expanding knowledge of deep venous disease.[8] Although deep venous treatment is not the subject of this work, a few concepts from the UIP document should be appreciated by those performing duplex of the lower extremity venous system:

- Iliac vein obstruction is ubiquitous and often silent in the general population.
- C3–C6 patients with primary and post-thrombotic chronic venous insufficiency (CVI), >90 percent with IVUS.
- Early restoration of iliac vein patency in the acute phase is becoming the norm to prevent post-thrombotic syndrome.
- Failure of the extremity to thrive following correction of superficial reflux is an indication for deep vein reconstruction.

In conclusion, venous testing is available in both direct and indirect testing modalities. Radiographic and more invasive methods can be complementary. The specific indications for use and application should be understood by clinicians with an interest in phlebology. Most importantly, understanding the limitations and information that can be gained with these various techniques will influence decision making in the treatment paradigm for the patients in our care.

Table 3.2 Air plethysmography study criteria.

	Normal	SVI	DVI	DVO
VFI	<2 mL/sec	2–20 (average 4)	4–25 (11)	3–20 (8)
EF	>60%	30–75%	20–55%	18–50%
RV	<35%	35%	>35%	>35%

DVI, deep venous insufficiency; DVO, deep venous obstruction; EF, ejection fraction; RV, residual venous; SVI, superficial venous insufficiency; VFI, venous refilling index.

REFERENCES

1. Marston WA, Wells-Brabham V, Mendes R *et al.* The importance of deep venous reflux velocity as a determination of outcome in patients with combined superficial and deep venous reflux treated with endovenous saphenous ablation. *Journal of Vascular Surgery* 2008; **48**: 400–6.

2. Marston WA, Owens LV, Davies S *et al.* Endovenous saphenous ablation corrects the hemodynamic abnormality in patients with CEAP clinical class 3-6 CVI due to superficial reflux. *Vascular and Endovascular Surgery* 2006; **40**: 125–30.

3. Bergan J. *The vein book.* Burlington, MA: Elsevier Academic Press, 2007.

4. Goldman M, Bergan J, Gues JJ. *Sclerotherapy: treatment of varicose and telangiectatic leg veins*, 4th edn. Philadelphia, PA: Mosby, Elsevier, 2007.

5. Meissner M, Moneta G, Burnand K *et al.* The hemodynamics and diagnosis of venous disease. *Journal of Vascular Surgery* 2007; **46**: 4S–24S.

6. Needham T. Assessment of lower extremity venous valvular insufficiency examinations. *Journal of Vascular Ultrasound* 2005; **29**: 123–9.

7. Park U-J, Yun W-S, Lee K-B *et al.* Analysis of the postoperative hemodynamic changes in varicose vein surgery using air plethysmography. *Journal of Vascular Surgery* 2010; **51**: 634–8.

8. Lurie F, Kistner R, Perrin M *et al.* Invasive treatment of deep venous disease, a UIP consensus. *International Angiology* 2010; **29**: 199–204.

4

Practical start-up tips for image optimization and acquisition

This chapter is intended to provide foundational information for those who are relatively new to ultrasound, but also suggestions and tips for the experienced sonographer that may prove of benefit with time-saving suggestions and improved techniques.

For the beginner, understanding how the transducer and monitor are related is a key fundamental. One needs to understand that the ultrasound beam is emitted out of the probe. The field of view that is created extends from the probe. In Figure 4.1, the area under the probe designates the field of view.

For visual relationships, Figure 4.2 demonstrates how the ultrasound (US) beam relates to the field of view on the monitor that displays information.

Once the way in which the ultrasound beam extends from the probe is understood, the image created on the monitor is as well. As the probe is placed on the body, the field of view looks into the body, allowing us to examine the area which is directly under the ultrasound probe. We must also appreciate that the ultrasound beam is extremely narrow when viewed on end, or along the long axis of the probe; this helps us to understand that the image displayed on the monitor represents only a very thin slice of information located directly along the axis of the ultrasound beam (Figure 4.3).

Although the images above provide for fundamental concepts of image acquisition and display, understanding image orientation in this matter will also help you understand how the image relates to the anatomy displayed, and to any ultrasound-guided applications.

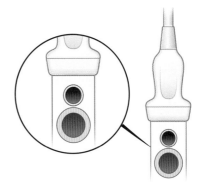

Figure 4.1 Ultrasound beam.

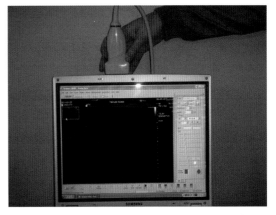

Figure 4.2 Relationship between the ultrasound beam and the field of view on the monitor.

Transducer/image orientation

Historically, ultrasound images have always been oriented so they are anatomically and radiographically

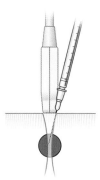

Figure 4.3 Narrow beam.

standardized. This concept is the same as with other imaging techniques, i.e. x-ray, computed tomography (CT) scan. By using a standard or universal approach, anyone viewing the images will appreciate the orientation and thus correctly understand the anatomic orientation. For anyone with no formal radiologic or image interpretation experience, this section is crucial.

As will be noted again below, ultrasound equipment cannot think, and only produces the image based upon what appears under the probe. Therefore, the orientation of the probe can have a significant impact on the image, and thus the understanding or interpretation of the image obtained. From a practical standpoint, flipping the probe 180° would produce mirror images of the same information (Figure 4.4).

The two main anatomic views in vascular ultrasound imaging are: (1) transverse (short axis), and (2) longitudinal (sagittal). Each approach has advantages and limitations. By understanding and using both approaches, important anatomic information can be gathered and correctly interpreted.

Transverse or short axis divides the body cross-sectionally into top (superior) and bottom (inferior) sections (Figure 4.5). From a practical standpoint, this means that images are like a slice horizontally through the body. In Figure 4.6, note that the femoral artery and vein, which are running from the feet towards the trunk of the body appear as circles in the image. In this orientation, the cross-section or short axis image of the artery and vein are presented. The photo on the left shows how the probe is placed on the leg, and the duplex image on the right demonstrates the image format (transverse) (Figure 4.6).

A longitudinal or sagittal approach divides the body into right and left sections along a long or vertical axis. From a practical standpoint, this means that images are like a slice vertically through the body. In the images below, note that the same femoral artery and vein, which are running from the feet towards the trunk of the body, appear as elongated tubes across the image. Again see how the probe is placed on the leg, and the image that is produced (Figure 4.7).

When scanning in transverse, medial is to the right on the screen (vein to the right of the artery) on the right leg. Conversely, medial is to the left on the screen on the left leg.

Example

On the right leg, the great saphenous vein (GSV) is medial (on the right side of the screen) to the common femoral vein (CFV) and common femoral artery (CFA). On the left leg, the GSV is medial (on the left side of the screen) to the CFV and CFA (Figure 4.8).

When scanning in the longitudinal axis, proximal or central (patient's head) is to the left, distal or peripheral (patient's feet) is to the right on the ultrasound image. This is the same for both the right and left legs. Therefore, when going from transverse to longitudinal, just turn the transducer to the right (clockwise) by 90°.

TIP All transducers have some kind of 'raised marker' to indicate one end of the long axis of the beam. Always keep the raised marker at 9 o'clock when scanning in transverse and at 12 o'clock in longitudinal.

Figure 4.9a,b shows the 9 and 12 o'clock position of the probe, which is simply accomplished with clockwise rotation.

Holding the transducer

When in the transverse approach, the more perpendicular you are to the vessel being imaged, the sharper your image. In Figure 4.10, image (a) on the left, will produce a sharper, clearer image. If you tilt the probe at an angle, as in image (b), there will be a suboptimal image produced.

(a)   (b)

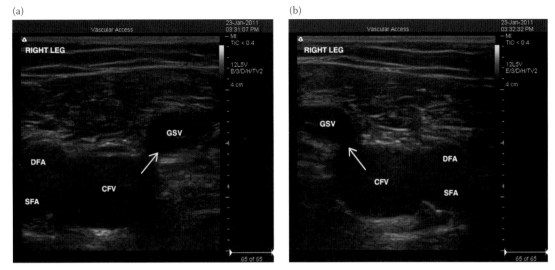

Figure 4.4 Duplex image showing mirror image produced by rotation of the probe by 180° – note the relation of the GSV to the CFV in each image (a and b).

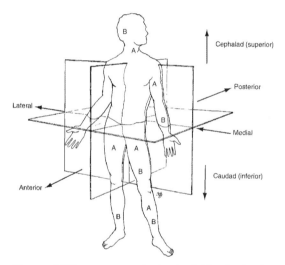

Figure 4.5 Transverse or short axis divides the body cross-sectionally into top (superior) and bottom (inferior) sections.

A common problem for sonographers who are new to superficial vein work has to do with probe pressure. In carrying out deep venous evaluations, every segment of the vein is imaged (Figures 4.11 and 4.12) with a normal image and one that is compressed showing vein wall coaptation.

This inherently 'trains' the technologist to increase their hand pressure, since they always need to scan deep veins and compress them. However, when scanning superficial veins, lighter pressure will give

(a)

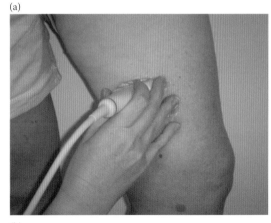

(b)

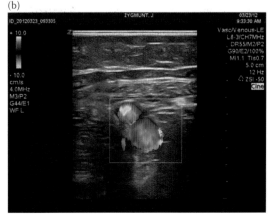

Figure 4.6 a,b Transverse image approach.

(a)

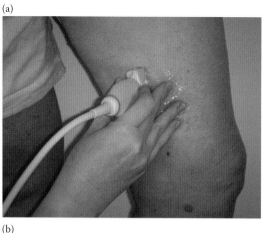

(b)

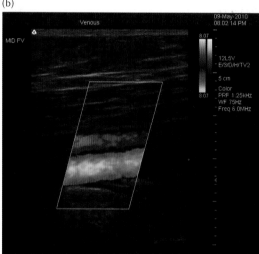

Figure 4.7 a,b Long axis approach.

(a)

(b)

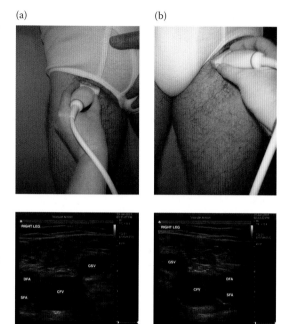

Figure 4.8 a,b When scanning in transverse, medial is to the right on the screen (vein to the right of the artery) in the right leg. Conversely, medial is to the left on the screen on the left leg.

a better image. The technologist should not press too hard as this risks collapsing, or partially collapsing, the vein. A heavy hand will make a vein appear smaller on the screen, and in some cases may bring valve leaflets closer together. In order to avoid this, you can help support the transducer by placing your little finger lightly on the skin (Figure 4.13). The finger becomes a gauge giving feedback regarding your probe pressure. If you are doing this correctly, your fingers will get a little messy with gel. Grasp the transducer so that you can make small adjustments with just the tips of your fingers. This is similar to how one holds a pencil, which is near the tip, to make micro-adjustments for writing, and using contact with the hand and the paper as a reference

point. If, however, one held a pencil near the eraser, fine motor control would be much harder.

When performing compression maneuvers, make the movements firm, deliberate, and smooth. A common mistake is to bounce the transducer on the leg when performing compressions. Unfortunately, a quicker bounce-type movement will not adequately show complete vein coaptation. A slow deliberate compression should be made (Figure 4.14). If a probe bounce is performed too quickly, an incomplete coaptation could be done and a situation as noted in this image may be falsely called negative, because the bounce was too quick and coaptation assumed and not actually visualized.

'Heel and toe' technique

When using Doppler (color or spectral) in a longitudinal axis, angle the vessel across the image to optimize the Doppler shift. Color Doppler will give a better fill of the vessel and spectral Doppler will give a better waveform.

(a)

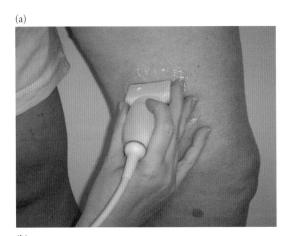

(b)

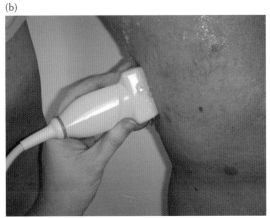

Figure 4.9 The 9 o'clock (a) and 12 o'clock (b) position of the probe on the leg.

(a)   (b)

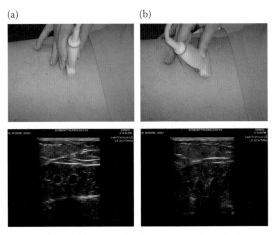

Figure 4.10 (a) Perpendicular versus (b) angled axis of probe with corresponding duplex image, note the sharper definition in the non-angled approach.

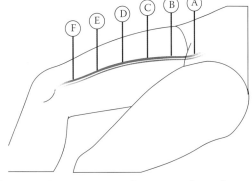

Figure 4.11 Deep compressions are performed every 1–2 cm.

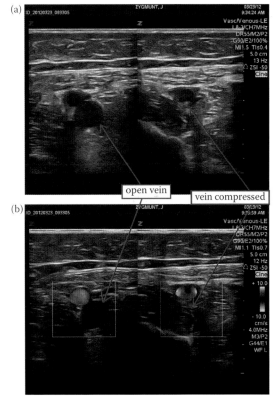

Figure 4.12 Split screen of duplex with compression shown in gray scale (a), and color (b). Note the color filling of the artery, with the vein below the artery.

To perform the 'heel and toe' technique (Figure 4.15), imagine one end of the transducer as the heel and the other end as the toe. Now put more pressure on one end of the probe, while allowing the other end to rest just off the skin surface.

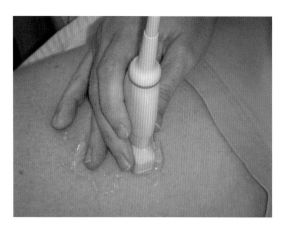

Figure 4.13 Fingers extended as guide with little finger in gel.

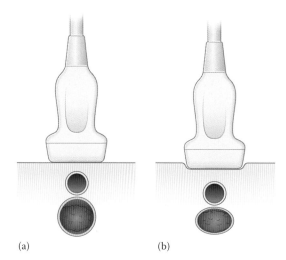

Figure 4.14 Probe without (left) and with compression (right), intraluminal thrombus is noted by incomplete compression of the (red) vein.

Ultrasound-guided procedures

Place the transducer and the patient in the best position possible. For instance, this may mean placing the patient in a sleeping position (Figure 4.16). Hold the transducer perpendicular (at a 90° angle) to the skin and make sure the darkest part of the vein is across as much of the screen as possible. Again be sure to use a light touch so you do not accidently collapse the vein. In Figure 4.16, the long axis approach will be used for an ultrasound-guided approach. The 90° approach on the left facilitates the ease of approach.

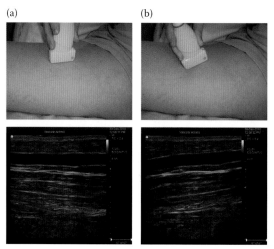

Figure 4.15 Heel and toe probe adjustment.

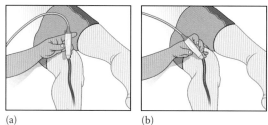

(a)   (b)

Figure 4.16 Optimal angle for ultrasound guidance on the left (a), while (b) is suboptimal.

'Knobology'

Most machines have presets for the various studies. Image picture quality (smoothness, graininess, contrast, etc.) is very subjective. Manufacturers recognize this and preload settings which help to optimize the image based on the depth of the image and other factors. The authors recommend starting with the appropriate preset for the study you want to perform and then making minor adjustments as needed. If you find yourself making the same adjustments repetitively to optimize your image, most systems will allow you to save your personal presets under a user profile, so these too can be loaded with the touch of a button, reducing the number of manual adjustments made during repetitive examinations.

The basic components and controls are the same on all the ultrasound machines. To make it easier to understand and refer to, we will divide this section into which knobs control the various ultrasound functions: B-mode controls, PWD (pulsed wave Doppler) controls, and color controls.

B-mode controls

B-mode stands for brightness mode and can be referred to as two-dimensional imaging.

- **Screen/monitor**. Adjust brightness/contrast, according to whether the room is bright or dark. This should be performed prior to adjusting the gain.
- **Overall (master) gain**. Used to increase or decrease the amount of amplification of returning echoes which effects the brightening or darkening of the image (Figure 4.17).
- **Time gain compensation (TGC)**. Controls the amount of gain in the image at different depths up or down in the field of view; balances the image to equalize the brightness of echoes from the near field to the far field (Figure 4.18).
- **Focus**. Used to optimize the image by increasing the resolution for a specific area; the focal zone should be placed at or just below the object of interest to achieve the sharpest image (Figure 4.19).
- **Depth**. Adjusts the field of view; increase to see larger or deeper structures (Figure 4.20).
- **Smoothing**. How smooth the image appears; more or less contrast.
- **Persistence**. Image frame averaging; if persistence is high, image appears less speckled and smoother.
- **Measurement**. Used to determine vessel diameter or percentage stenosis (Figure 4.21).

Pulsed wave Doppler controls

PWD is a series of pulses used to study the motion of blood flow. The x-axis represents time and the y-axis represents Doppler frequency shift. The velocity can be displayed as cm/s or kHz.

- **Sweep speed**. How fast the spectral waveforms move across the screen (slow to fast); set slow to medium for venous scanning.
- **Pulse repetition frequency**. Defines the velocity range of the display; should be set high enough to prevent aliasing, but low enough to provide adequate detection of slow blood flow (aliasing occurs when the frequency of

(a)
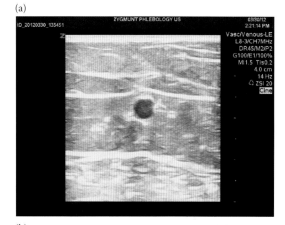

(b)
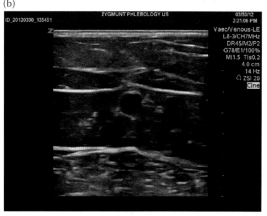

Figure 4.17 Duplex of image with over (too much) gain (a) and the proper amount of gain (b).

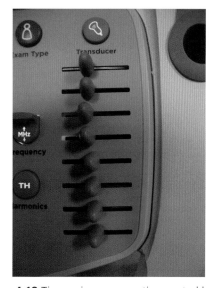

Figure 4.18 Time gain compensation control knobs.

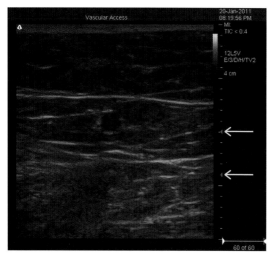

Figure 4.19 Focus zone with line indicator added.

what you are observing exceeds one half of the sample rate).

TIP Set at 1.2–1.5 kHz for venous scanning.

- **Wall filter.** Eliminates unwanted low frequency, high-intensity signals (also known as clutter):
  - Use a wall filter that is high enough to remove clutter, but low enough to display information near the baseline. An inappropriate setting will 'filter' out important information, especially when it comes to detecting slow flow venous reflux.

TIP Should be set low, usually 40–60 Hz is recommended for venous scanning.

- **Steering angle.** Used to maintain a Doppler angle of 60° or less.
- **Baseline (Doppler scale).** Allows you to move the baseline up or down and the change the scale of the Doppler display based on the various sizes of the waveforms. Data above represents flow towards the probe; data below represents flow away from the probe.
- **Correction angle.** Should be set at 60°; parallel to the vessel wall when performing venous studies.
- **Sample volume.** SV adjusts the size of the pulsed wave Doppler region being examined; displayed as two parallel lines (the distance between the lines is the size of the SV in mm).

(a)

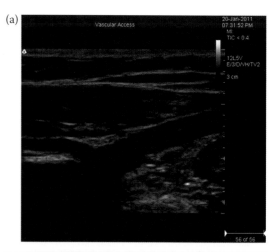

(b)

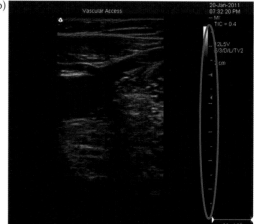

(c)

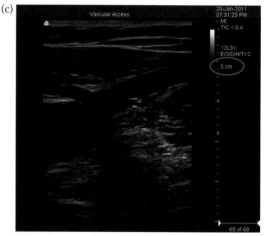

Figure 4.20 Depth shows at three different levels. This adjustment needs to be optimized for each image acquired. 5 cm as noted in image (c) is an appropriate scale.

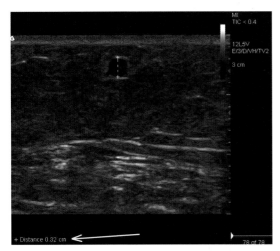

Figure 4.21 Duplex of calipers showing vein being measured.

For venous scanning, it should fit inside the vessel and not touch the vessel walls.

- **Gain.** Increases or decreases the amplification of the returning signal; gain should be adjusted so the spectral waveform is bright.

Color controls

Detects the presence, direction, and relative velocity of blood flow.

- **Steering angle.** An adequate Doppler angle-to-flow is required in order to obtain useful color Doppler information (Figure 4.22):
  - 90°, an absent or confusing color pattern is displayed
  - 60° or less is best.

TIP The 'heel and toe' technique can be used (using pressure on one end of the transducer or the other to improve the Doppler angle to flow).

- **Color flow box.** Controls the color sampling area; size should be just big enough to surround the vessel; angle the box at 45–60° to the vessel wall when evaluating the vein longitudinally, and 90° to the vessel wall when in transverse for a good Doppler shift (Figure 4.23).
- **Pulse repetition frequency.** Defines the velocity range of the display; should be set high enough

(a) 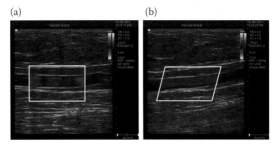 (b)

Figure 4.22 Steering of color box: (a) suboptimal angle and (b) better color box steering.

(a)
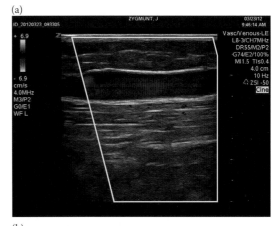

(b)
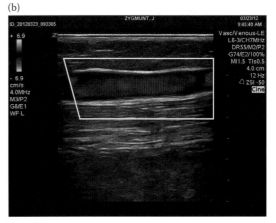

Figure 4.23 Color box too large (a) and one adjusted appropriately (b).

to prevent aliasing, but low enough to provide adequate detection of slow blood flow. Aliasing occurs when the frequency of what you are observing exceeds one half of the sample rate (Figure 4.24).

TIP 1.2–1.5 kHz is recommended for venous scanning.

(a)

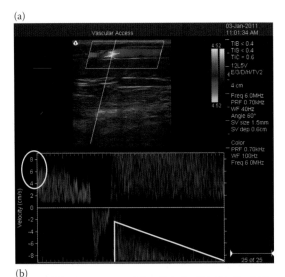

(b)

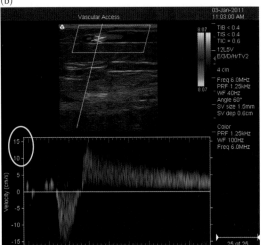

Figure 4.24 Aliasing duplex of venous flow (a) and a spectral image with correction to prevent aliasing (b).

■ **Wall filter**. Eliminates unwanted low frequency, high-intensity signals (also known as clutter). (Use a wall filter that is high enough to remove clutter, but low enough to display information near the baseline.)

TIP Should be set low, usually 40–60 Hz is recommended for venous scanning.

■ **Color priority**. Amount of color displayed over bright echoes; helps confine color within the vessel walls.
■ **Color persistence**. Determines the amount to be averaged between frames. Increased

persistence causes color to persist on the two-dimensional image, decreased persistence helps in the better detection of short detection jets.

■ **Color threshold**. Level of low velocity data displayed.
■ **Color gain**. Controls the strength of the signal displayed. If you have too much gain, there will be artifact, whereas if you have too little gain, you may miss slow flow (Figure 4.25).

TIP Try adjusting the gain slightly too high (when there is a great deal of speckling) then reduce the gain to where there are little to no speckles.

(a)

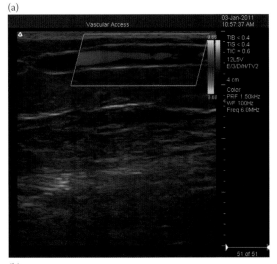

(b)

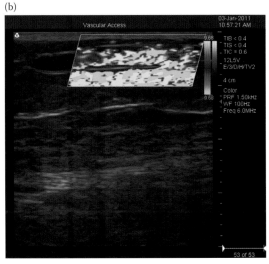

Figure 4.25 Color gain with image displayed correctly (a) and with the color gain too high below (b).

- **Invert**. Allows you to switch the direction of the color; making red flow blue and blue flow red.

TIP Remember the top of the color bar indicates blood flow towards the probe and the bottom of the color bar indicates blood flow away from the probe. When performing venous insufficiency studies, it is best to have red on the top and blue on the bottom since flow towards the probe would indicate reflux (red) when performing distal augmentation.

In conclusion, producing optimal ultrasound images is a skill that is developed over time, with a great deal of practice. Presented here are several key concepts which will help to further understand the process, with tips to help in various methods. This is not intended to be an exhaustive list of these topics, but is a foundation on which to build. In later chapters, these points and others may be described as specific protocols, and pathology and findings are discussed.

Special addendum for ultrasound-guided vein access procedures

The following pages outline the two main approaches for venous access using ultrasound guidance – long axis and short axis. These step-by-step pages demonstrate key points of the technique of ultrasound imaging which can be invaluable to the clinician learning ultrasound guidance. They are being provided in this special addendum as additional material to the information previously presented in this chapter.

Addendum

Vein access, transverse approach

1) Have the patient positioned in reverse Trendelenburg for better vein filling. Know the depth of the vein and the length of the access needle (2.75 inches or 7 cm).

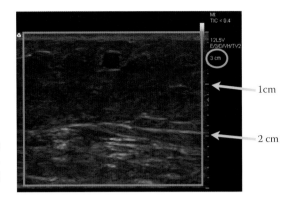

In the image above, the total depth of the image is 3 cm (see orange square). This information is available on the right side of the image (see orange circle). Each of the longer lines on the right side of the image denotes 1 cm (see green arrows), so the depth of the vein shown above is only 0.5 cm.

2) Position the vein in the center of the transducer.

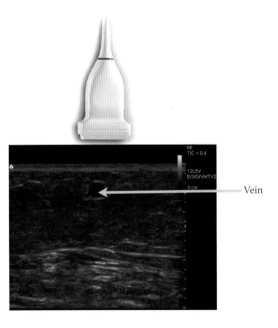

3) Ask the physician to inject a small amount (0.5 cc) of 1 percent lidocaine very superficially to create a skin wheal. Caution physician against injecting too much lidocaine because it may cause the vein to spasm. This can be done while the transducer is on the

skin so the physician knows the exact location for the lidocaine.

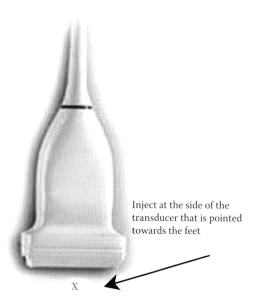

Inject at the side of the transducer that is pointed towards the feet

X

4) Have the physician/sonographer angle the transducer slightly toward the needle.

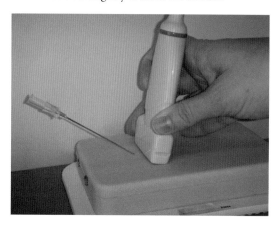

5) There are two approaches when accessing in transverse.

   a. The physician can come in with the needle (bevel up) at an almost perpendicular (straight up and down) approach with the transducer (see below), or

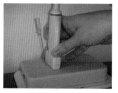

   b. The physician can come in with the needle (bevel up) at a less steep angle with the transducer (see below).

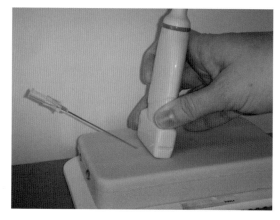

TIP Remember that you are not going to see the needle until it is under the ultrasound transducer.

6) Look for the needle tip to show up on the ultrasound image. This should appear as a bright white echo. Note whether the needle is medial or lateral to the target vein.

Medial 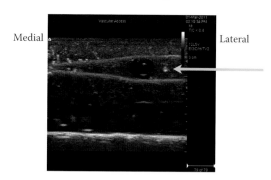 Lateral

In this example, the needle is lateral to the vein. Also note whether the needle is superficial or deep to the vein.

TIP If you are having trouble visualizing the needle tip on the ultrasound image, check to see how much of the length of the needle is in the leg. Remember you already noted the depth of the vein before the physician began. If most of the needle is in the leg and the vein was only 0.5–1 cm deep, then you need to instruct the physician to pull back because the needle tip is too deep (see below). To determine if the needle tip is below the vein, move the transducer cephalad (toward the patient's head) and try to visual the needle tip. Have the physician 'wiggle' the needle slightly so it is more easily visualized. Once the needle tip is located, the physician can start to slowly pull the needle out while sliding the transducer slowly back towards the needle.

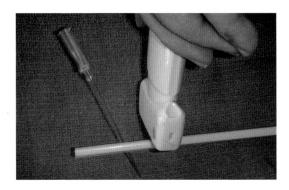

7) Instruct the physician on the location of the needle tip and offer instruction on how to move the needle or the hand of the physician to get the needle directly over the vein. For example, if the needle is lateral to the vein, ask the physician to slowly remove the needle and move slightly more medial along the transducer and try again.

TIP Prior to the physician using the needle, use a skin marker tip and 'poke' at the area of entry to determine the best location to enter.

8) Look for 'tenting' of the vein wall. This is where the top wall of the vein folds in when the needle is pushed against it.

9) When you see 'tenting' of the vein wall, instruct the physician to push through the vein wall. Remember the first attempt is the best attempt. Explain that they should feel a 'pop' once they are through. Look for blood return in the needle hub.

TIP If the physician feels they are in the vein but does not see any blood return, try to visualize the needle tip with ultrasound.

- The tip of the needle may be against the back wall of the vein. Instruct the physician to slowly pull back the needle while looking for blood return.
- Try 'twisting/turning' the needle to make sure the bevel of the needle is not against the vein wall.
- The physician can try attaching a syringe to the hub of the needle and try to aspirate. Although this can sometimes cause the physician to pull the needle out of the vein.

If there is no blood return it may be that the needle has 'slipped' off the vein and is to the side. In this case, the physician should reposition the needle over the top of the vein again, look for the 'tenting', and try again.

10) Another method for vein access is called the 'double wall puncture'. This involves directing the needle through the top and bottom walls of the vein. Once the needle is through both vein walls, the physician pulls back the needle slowly and looks for the bottom wall of the vein to 'drop' off the needle tip (see below). At that point, the physician should see blood return in the needle hub.

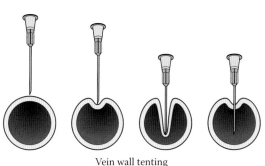

Vein wall tenting

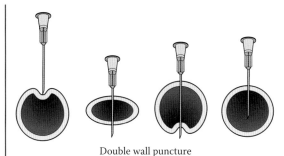

Double wall puncture

TIP If the physician is getting flashback, but cannot advance the guidewire, try changing into the longitudinal view so that the needle is visualized inside the vein. This allows the physician to see if the needle tip is against the back wall of the vein. Then the physician can reposition the needle tip either by pulling back slightly, so the tip is located more in the center of the vein lumen, or by pressing the needle hub towards the patient's skin allowing the needle tip to detach from the vein wall.

Longitudinal approach

1) Have the patient positioned in reverse Trendelenburg for better vein filling. Know the depth of the vein and the length of the access needle (2.75 in or 7 cm).

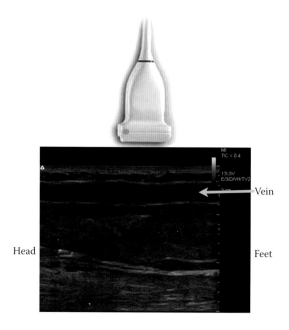

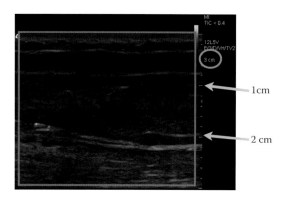

In the image above, the total depth of the image is 3 cm (see orange square). This information is available on the right side of the image (see orange circle). Each of the longer lines on the right side of the image denotes 1 cm (see green arrows), so the depth of the vein shown above is only 0.5 cm.

2) Position the widest and darkest part of the vein across the entire length of the screen.

3) Ask the physician to inject a small amount (0.5 cc) of 1 percent lidocaine (plain) very superficially to create a skin wheal. Caution physician against injecting too much lidocaine because it may cause the vein to spasm. This can be done while the transducer is on the skin so the physician knows the exact location for the lidocaine.

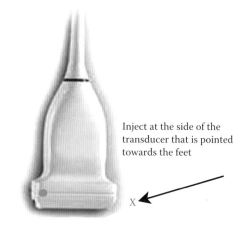

Inject at the side of the transducer that is pointed towards the feet

4) Have the physician/sonographer hold the transducer perpendicular (90° angle to the skin), not tilted to one side.

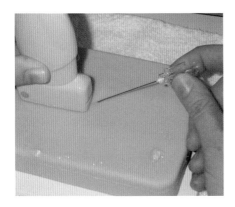

TIP Make sure the physician lines up the needle (bevel up) directly in the center of the end of the transducer and does not have the needle enter at too steep an angle with the transducer. Instead, angle the needle slightly so the tip of the needle will travel under the transducer. The angle of the needle depends on the depth of the vein. If the vein is only 1 cm deep use a shallow angle (15–30°), whereas if the vein is 2–3 cm deep, you will have to use a steeper angle. Try not to exceed an angle of 45°. Remember that you are not going to see the needle until it is under the ultrasound transducer.

5) Look for the needle length to enter the field. This should appear as a bright white echo. The more clearly you see the entire length of the needle, the better you are lined up with the vein for access. Also note whether the needle is superficial or deep to the vein.

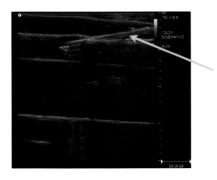

TIP If the physician is having trouble seeing the needle, look at his hand and the needle in relation to the transducer. The needle should be parallel to the transducer, not angled to the side.

(a) 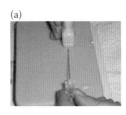   (b)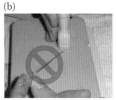

6) Instruct the physician on the location of the needle and offer instruction on how to move the needle or the hand of the physician to get the needle in line with the transducer. With the longitudinal approach, you will be mostly looking at the alignment of the needle to the transducer (not the ultrasound image) to guide the physician. For example, if the needle is angled to the left of the transducer, ask the physician to slowly move the hub of the needle and his hand to the right so that the entire length of the needle is parallel to the transducer. The needle should appear on the screen.

(a) 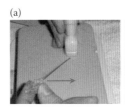   (b)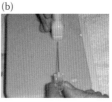

7) Once the needle is visualized on the screen, look for 'tenting' of the vein wall. This is where the top wall of the vein folds in when the needle is pushed against it.

(a) 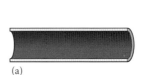   (b)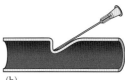

8) When you see 'tenting' of the vein wall, instruct the physician to push through the vein wall. Remember the first attempt is the best attempt. Explain that they should feel a 'pop' once they are through. Look for blood return in the needle hub.

TIP If the physician feels they are in the vein, but does not see any blood return, try to visualize the needle tip with ultrasound.

- The tip of the needle may be against the back wall of the vein. Instruct the physician to slowly pull back the needle while looking for blood return.
- Try moving your needle to one side and then the other. If you move the needle to the left and distort the image of the vein, then the vein must be to the left of the needle.
- The physician can try attaching a syringe to the hub of the needle and try to aspirate, although this can sometimes cause the physician to pull the needle out of the vein.

If there is no blood return it may be that the needle has 'slipped' off the vein and is to the side. In this case, the physician should reposition the needle over the top of vein again, look for the 'tenting' and try again.

9) Another method for vein access is called the 'double wall puncture'. This involves directing the needle through the top and bottom walls of the vein. Once the needle is through both vein walls, the physician pulls back the needle slowly and looks for the bottom wall of the vein to 'drop' off the needle tip. At that point, the physician should see blood return in the needle hub.

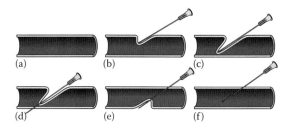

5

Practical guide to scanning, including the deep, small saphenous vein and great saphenous vein

Introduction

According to Virchow's triad, venous thrombosis occurs due to one of three factors: (1) decreased blood flow (stasis), (2) injury to the vessel wall, and (3) a hypercoagulable state. There are several independent risk factors for venous thromboembolism (VTE), including surgery, hospitalization, immobilization, prolonged bed rest, prolonged travel, smoking, obesity, age, use of oral contraceptives/hormones, pregnancy, varicose veins, and dehydration, among others. There are also medical conditions that can lead to VTE, including but not limited to: compression of the veins, recent trauma, cancer, infections, and heart disease.

Deep venous thrombosis (DVT) is estimated to affect 20–30 percent of all major surgical patients.[1] In general, DVT incidence in the United States is estimated at 600 000–2 000 000 events per year.[2] Further it is estimated that at least 50 000 and perhaps as many as 200 000 patients die from pulmonary embolism (PE) each year.[3] Interestingly, only 25 percent of patients with DVT display clinical signs of DVT[4] and, furthermore, that due to this asymptomatic nature, its initial presentation may be that of fatal PE.[5] A late complication of DVT is post-thrombotic syndrome (PTS) which can manifest itself as edema, pain or discomfort, and skin

problems, including venous ulceration. Although PTS was historically thought of as taking years to develop, recent thinking suggests that with major iliofemoral thrombosis, sequelae of PTS can present in as little as three years in 35–69 percent of cases.[6] Thus, the temporal meaning of the term 'late' is changing.

These statistics are staggering and only reinforce the importance of diagnosis of DVT, which is primarily done through duplex ultrasound. This section provides foundational information on duplex ultrasound and tips for its practical application for scanning the lower extremity venous system for DVT or chronic venous disease (CVD).

Ultrasound terms used when assessing veins

Echogenicity

Echogenicity relates to the ability to create an echo. When a vein is described as having a low level of echogenicity it means there are few echoes (bright areas) within the vein lumen. This could be because the vein is full of blood, or with acute (fresh) thrombus. Another word for no or low echogenicity is anechoic, meaning without echoes. Conversely, when a vein is described as having bright or high echogenicity (hyperechoic), it means there are many echoes or bright areas within the vein lumen. Hyperechoes typically indicate thrombosis within the vein lumen. With increasing chronicity (age), the characteristics of echogenicity increase. Most often, as the thrombus ages, there is increased fibrin organization, vein wall thickening, remodeling of the fibrous clot to collagen, and as all this begins to occur, so does atrophy of the vein wall and its diameter. Collagen is a higher reflector of ultrasound, thus a brighter echo (Figure 5.1).

Compressibility

Veins, in contrast to arteries, have thin walls and lower blood pressure, therefore veins can easily be collapsed with a relatively small amount of external pressure. Compressibility is the most reliable way of diagnosing intraluminal thrombus. A vein containing thrombus within it cannot be compressed even with considerable pressure. The compression technique is best performed in a transverse or short-axis view using gray scale. Figure 5.2 shows the open vein, compressed vein, and an artist rendering of venous compression.

Spontaneous flow

Large veins such as the inferior vena cava (IVC), iliac, femoral, and popliteal vessels demonstrate spontaneous blood flow when at rest. This flow reflects respiratory changes. For instance, if a patient lies still on the examination table and an ultrasound probe is placed on the femoral vein, you should see blood flow in gray scale with respiration. If you turn on spectral Doppler and place the sample volume within the femoral vein lumen, a spectral waveform should be recorded. If you turn on color Doppler and place the color box over the femoral vein, you

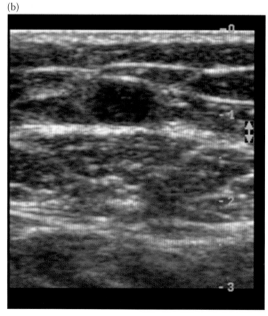

Figure 5.1 (a) The vein is anechoic, however, in (b) there are increased echoes within the lumen.

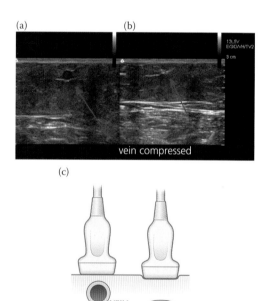

Figure 5.2 The vein is open in (a) (see arrow) and compressed in (b) the diagrams show this in (c).

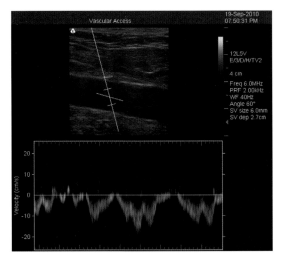

Figure 5.3 Spontaneous spectral flow in the common femoral vein.

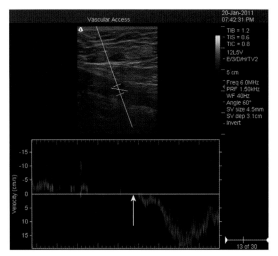

Figure 5.4 To the left of the arrow, the patient is holding his breath showing the lack of venous flow, which returns to the right of the arrow upon exhalation.

should see intermittent color fill the lumen of the femoral vein. Smaller veins and veins more distally located, such as the calf veins, usually do not produce spontaneous flow due to their size, the slow velocity of flow within them, and distance from these thoracoabdominal effects. Absence of spontaneous flow could indicate an obstruction either central (proximal) or peripheral (distal) to the area you are examining. This is one of the key criteria used in diagnosis of venous flow. One should also be aware of the effect position has on this criteria, i.e. this should be evaluated in the supine or slight tilt position, not the standing position (Figure 5.3).

Phasic flow

Normal venous flow is phasic, which means that the velocity of flow changes in response to respiration. As noted above, this can be demonstrated with spectral and color Doppler. Normal flow stops during inspiration and returns during expiration. This is because with inspiration, the diaphragm moves down and increases intra-abdominal pressure. This increase in pressure puts external force on the IVC and iliac veins, slowing venous return from the legs. With expiration, the diaphragm moves up and the intra-abdominal pressure reduces, allowing for increased flow from the legs into the iliacs and IVC. As noted before, there are many things which can

affect the spectral signal. For instance, a continuous flow pattern suggests there may be obstruction central to the site being examined.[7] Remember that if the thrombus is not completely occlusive, there still may be phasic signals, therefore phasic signals do not exclude a thrombus. These changes can be quite subtle. Figure 5.4 demonstrates the changes that occur with a patient holding their breath.

Augmentation

Augmentation is a provoked maneuver used to evaluate the venous system. By applying a moderately firm squeeze over the calf, a wave of venous flow is created that leaves the calf in a central direction. This 'augmentation' causes an increase in flow moving central in normal veins. This maneuver is used to confirm patency of the vein segment between the site of the Doppler probe and the site of calf compression. If the augmentation signal is crisp and clean, the assumption is that the vein is clear. However, if the signal is blunted or muted in some way, this suggests obstruction which could be either intra- or extravascular.

For insufficiency examinations, we also use augmentation as a systolic maneuver, and upon release of a distal augmentation in a normal vein, we typically do not hear flow. If, however, we hear backflow after the release of an augmentation maneuver, this indicates reflux. This is the diastolic phase. Although this will be covered more fully later in this chapter, the reader should be aware that augmentation can test both patency and valvular function.

Valsalva maneuver

The Valsalva maneuver is a provoked maneuver which is used to stress the venous system and evaluate flow characteristics. When properly done, the patient would take a breath in, and while holding the breath, exert pressure by 'bearing down' as if simulating a bowel movement or an abdominal crunch. This causes an increase of intra-abdominal pressure with the primary goal of testing the flow characteristics and valve functions in the central (proximal) vessels. This downward pressure is typically transmitted down and through non-functioning valves until it reaches *the first competent valve*. Unfortunately, this information is not universally understood by those performing venous ultrasound and is therefore stressed. Once a competent valve is encountered, the pressure wave stops being transmitted distally. In this manner, if a common femoral vein is competent (normal), the Valsalva maneuver will not adequately test the femoral vein valves (or any distal valves) for competency. Proper patient instruction is critical for this test to be of value – as often patients do not perform this test adequately. There are several methods that can be used for this. One would be to place a hand on the patient's stomach and ask them to 'push out' against the hand. A second would be to have the patient place a thumb in their mouth, and pretend this is a balloon to be blown up – each of these maneuvers produce the same intra-abdominal increase in pressure to properly test venous function.

More recently, a standardized method using a measuring tube was described by De Maeseneer and colleagues.[8] The approach, while standardized, appears to be cumbersome, and may have limited adoption.

Sonographic features of normal veins

In gray scale or B-mode, a normal vein has a thin, smooth wall with an anechoic lumen with no intraluminal echoes. Normal veins are fully compressible

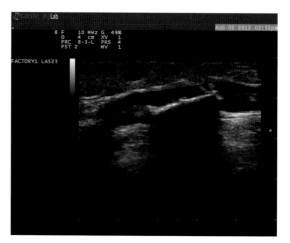

Figure 5.5 Chronic venous thrombosis with shadow.

with probe compression. When using spectral Doppler, there is spontaneous, phasic flow in the larger deep veins which augment with distal compression. Color Doppler demonstrates complete color filling of the lumen with a phasic pattern.

Sonographic features of abnormal veins

In gray scale or B-mode, an abnormal vein has an echogenic lumen which may be partially or fully non-compressible (Figure 5.5). If the vein is occluded it may appear distended, especially in the acute phase of thrombosis. Spectral Doppler may be near normal or abnormal depending on the extent of the thrombus load. A continuous Doppler signal or a Doppler signal with absent or reduced phasicity could indicate an obstruction. Absence of a spectral Doppler signal or color Doppler signal would indicate a total obstruction. Be careful when using color Doppler since it may not be accurate if the controls are not adjusted properly, and a false positive may be suggested.

Characterizing thrombus (acute versus chronic)

Acute thrombus

Identifying the age of a thrombus can prove difficult. Signs that a thrombus is acute (first 14 days) include: (1) the thrombosed vein is usually distended and larger than the adjacent artery; (2) has low echogenicity and may be anechoic; (3) appears 'spongy' or deforms slightly with probe pressure, but remains either partially or completely non-compressible; and (4) the proximal end is often not attached to the vein wall, but 'floats' in the lumen.

When an acute thrombus is identified, especially when the thrombus is free floating, proceed with caution in order to avoid dislodging the thrombus during the examination. The extent of the thrombus should be evaluated with as little manipulation as possible. This could be a life-threatening finding, and in most settings, established protocols would include immediate notification of the interpreting physician, the ordering physician and an urgent trip to the emergency department. Newer procedures are slowly being adopted for the removal of thrombus load during the first 30 days after onset. Current thinking is that removal of the thrombus load, with for instance a Trellis™ peripheral infusion system, prevention of damage to the valves, and early restoration of patency will greatly reduce the development and severity of PTS, following DVT.

Chronic thrombus

Signs that a thrombus is chronic include: (1) a high echogenicity; (2) contracted in size; usually the vein is the same or smaller size than the artery; (3) large collateral veins are often present; (4) flow can be seen in areas of recanalization; (5) the vein walls are thickened; and (6) the presence of webbing in the vein lumen.

Documentation, suggestions and tips

Duplex ultrasonography is used to assess the anatomy and physiology of the deep and superficial venous system of the lower extremities. As described earlier, duplex has two parts, each providing complementary information to the other. Gray-scale or B-mode imaging is used in the detection, location, and characterization of venous anatomy, structure, and pathology, and also provides information about soft tissues and surrounding structures. Venous hemodynamics are evaluated using Doppler signals. Spectral Doppler analysis provides quantitative information about hemodynamic blood flow. Color flow Doppler is the third part of the equation,

sometimes referred to as Tri-Plex, and provides Doppler information in another format. This also provides quantitative information about hemodynamics of the blood flow.

Below the reader will find helpful information regarding practical steps used to perform duplex ultrasound examination. The information presented comes not only from the practical experience of the authors, but also from guidelines and suggestions from some leading medical societies or organizations in the United States, including but not limited to:

American College of Phlebology (ACP)[9]
Society of Vascular Ultrasound (SVU)[10]
American College of Radiology (ACR) (joint statement with American Institute of Ultrasound in Medicine (AIUM) and Society of Radiologists in Ultrasound (SRU))[11]
Intersocietal Commission on the Accreditation of Vascular Laboratories (ICAVL)[12]

Immediately following these will be sample forms which may prove helpful for anyone just starting out in the field. More information and sample protocols will appear in Chapter 6. This foundational section provides the backdrop and methodologies upon which these protocols can be performed.

Indications for peripheral venous ultrasound examinations may include, but are not limited to the following conditions/situations:

1. Evaluation of possible venous obstruction or thrombus or thromboembolic disease in symptomatic or high-risk asymptomatic individuals.
2. Assessment of venous insufficiency and its related signs and symptoms, i.e. venous varicosities, venous ulcer, pain, edema, venous stasis, etc., including pretreatment vein mapping for the phlebology patient.
3. Assessment of calf muscle pump function.
4. Assessment of dialysis access grafts.
5. Venous mapping prior to harvest for arterial bypass or reconstructive surgery.
6. Evaluation of veins prior to venous access.
7. Evaluation for DVT in patients with suspected pulmonary embolism.
8. Follow up for patients with known venous thrombosis.

9. Status post-venous interventional procedure.
10. A palpable cord.

Contraindications and limitations include, but are not limited to:

1. Obesity
2. Casts, dressings, open wounds, etc. (exceptions noted)
3. Severe edema, and
4. Limited patient mobility and inability to stand.

For ease of performance, establish a good rapport with the patient. Before beginning any examination, always introduce yourself to the patient and briefly explain what you are about to do. This will help alleviate any anxiety the patient may have about the examination. Be sure to mention that the examination is non-invasive and explain what they are going to feel (gel, pressure, calf squeezing, etc.). Since a physician has to interpret the examination,[13] a sonographer should not answer questions related to their specific diagnosis, instead refer them to their physician for answers. It is also noted that there are specific protocols for duplex venous ultrasound for DVT and for chronic venous insufficiency (CVI), which although similar are not exactly the same. Table 5.1 presents the differences between these two protocols as described by ICAVL.[12]

Examination techniques for deep venous scanning

A short bullet-type document of this scanning technique is also provided at the end of this chapter.

Table 5.1 Differences between specific protocols for duplex venous ultrasound for deep vein thrombosis (DVT) and chronic venous insufficiency (CVI).

Transverse gray scale	Spectral wave forms
DVT protocol	
Common femoral vein, saphenofemoral junction	Right and left common femoral vein[7]
Proximal, mid, and distal femoral vein	
Popliteal vein	Popliteal vein
Post-tibial vein	
Peroneal vein	
Additional images as needed	
Additional as per protocol	Additional as per protocol
Reflux (CVI) protocol	
Common femoral vein	Common femoral vein (right/left)
Saphenofemoral junction	Saphenofemoral junction
Mid-femoral vein	Femoral vein
Great saphenous vein	Great saphenous vein (multiple sites[a])
Popliteal vein	Popliteal vein
Small saphenous vein	Small saphenous vein
Additional images as needed	Suspected areas of reflux[7]
Additional as per protocol	Additional as per protocol

Modified from ICAVL standards 2010.[12]

[a] Iliacs, great saphenous vein, small saphenous vein, proximal profunda, gastrocnemius veins, soleus veins, anterior tibials, perforators.

Patient assessment

Obtain a complete and pertinent medical history, including the relevant risk factors for lower extremity peripheral venous disease: previous deep vein and/or superficial vein thrombosis, trauma of the lower extremity, immobilization, recent major surgery, prolonged bed rest, history of cancer, family history of DVT, pregnancy, hypercoagulopathy, congestive heart failure or other cardiac disease, current medications, and results of other relevant diagnostic procedures.

Perform a limited physical examination which includes looking for any signs or symptoms of peripheral venous disease, such as swelling, pain, tenderness, palpable cord, discoloration, varicosities, and ulceration. The purpose of this is to key in on the patient's complaints so that we are able to determine if the ultrasound findings match the clinical condition of the patient.

Patient positioning

When scanning the deep system of the lower extremities, it is best to put the patient in the supine position and the examination table in a slight reverse Trendelenburg (10–20°). This helps blood to pool in the legs and therefore the veins will enlarge, making them easier to visualize on ultrasound, especially the calf veins. The patient's leg should be externally rotated with the knee slightly bent (Figure 5.6).

To examine the veins (deep or superficial) of the calf, the patient can also sit with the legs dangling over the side of the bed (Figure 5.7). Always remember, placing the patient in a dependent position will allow for venous filling which makes the veins easier to see and evaluate due to their increased size. The patient and the room should be warm to prevent vasoconstriction.

Also for evaluation of deep vein insufficiency, a steep tilt or standing position is best to test valve competency. Reflux concepts will be covered more fully in a later section of this chapter.

Equipment and probe selection

A high resolution ultrasound machine with real-time imaging, superior gray scale, an integrated pulsed, and range-gated Doppler is required. Many of today's ultrasound units offer variable frequency probes. Record keeping and storage is critical, therefore the ability to record the Doppler waveform and image is highly recommended. Most current ultrasound systems available today provide for video output in digital format which, along with most other medical records, is becoming the preferred format. At the end of a given study, a series of image prints of video clips should be stored for the interpreting physician to review and dictate the report. These digital prints need to be archived properly according to state or local laws regarding medical record storage.

A linear array transducer with a range of 5–8 MHz is typically recommended for evaluating

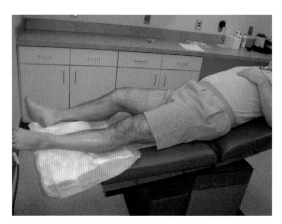

Figure 5.6 Typical patient positioning for DVT examination.

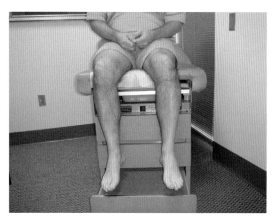

Figure 5.7 Patient positioning for evaluation of calf veins.

the deep venous system. You will need a lower frequency transducer in order to see the deep vessels in the thigh of some larger patients. In some situations, this may also require a curvilinear probe which has lower frequencies and depth penetration for patients with very large legs or to visualize the iliac veins. More recently, there is growing interest in iliac obstruction, stenting and resulting need for suprainguinal imaging. This is causing more of the curvilinear probes to be used either alone, or prior to magnetic resonance venography or even intravascular ultrasound (IVUS). There will be more on iliac scanning later in this chapter.

Examination techniques

Appropriate techniques need to be used to assess the presence and severity of any venous abnormalities. The entire lower extremity venous system should be assessed using both imaging and Doppler interrogation. These two formats provide different, yet complementary information regarding the status of the venous system and blood flow.

Using B-mode imaging, check for the compressibility of the vein, the walls of the vein should completely collapse or coapt. By applying external pressure slowly and evenly, a vein can be compressed until the two vein walls touch. This should be performed in gray scale using a transverse axis, not the longitudinal axis. Compression ultrasound findings are the main criteria to diagnose or exclude venous thrombosis. A common error is to bounce the probe during compression which may lead to a false negative. Be sure to make compressions with a slow deliberate motion bringing the walls into contact with each other. Typically, while performing this maneuver, the vein will coapt and the pulsatility of the corresponding artery is more easily seen.

Also note that this compression maneuver is performed approximately every 1–2 cm along the entire length of the vein being interrogated. In Figure 5.8, the serial compressions are made at locations A–F along the course of the veins of the deep thigh. This is a key point, in order to rule out DVT. A single compression at each of the common femoral vein (CFV), femoral vein (FV), or popliteal vein (PV) is insufficient. For completeness and

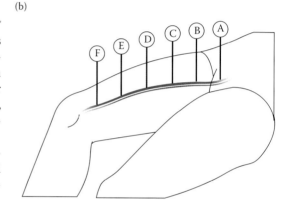

Figure 5.8 (a) The coaptation of a vein with external compression and (b) the typical locations for deep vein compression maneuvers in the thigh.

quality, interrogation along the course of the entire vein being examined is required.

If a vein fails to compress, as noted on the right side of Figure 5.8a, this could be due to intraluminal thrombus within the vein. *This is the most reliable method to diagnosis thrombosis.* Beware, however, that there are some areas in the leg in which performing a compression is difficult, such as the distal Hunterian canal. Due to the muscle structure in that area and how the vein moves into the popliteal space, it can be often difficult to see the vein in its entirety (near areas E and F in Figure 5.8b). In areas like this, a combination of characteristics is used, adding color flow and spectral flow analysis to the compression technique.

Using spectral Doppler, check for spontaneous, phasic flow and augmentation with distal compression, as well as for valve competence. Although this can be performed in duplex or triplex (color), for documentation purposes, be sure to obtain spectral waveforms in a longitudinal axis using a Doppler angle of 60° or less, and keep the cursor aligned parallel to the vessel wall. **Spectral analysis is like time delay photography in that the curve shows what takes place along a temporal window extending for several seconds. Static color flow images are not adequate to document reflux, since it will only show one instant in time and not allow for quantization of the reflux**. This key concept is also shown in Chapter 1 (Figure 1.13) and shows how the spectral curve has been 'colorized' to indicate when red or blue would appear on color flow as compared to the spectral curve. **This indicates why a 'flash' of red on a static image is non-diagnostic**.

Before beginning the scan, check the equipment gain and display settings to be sure they are optimized to provide the best possible B-mode, spectral, and/or color flow Doppler images. For venous studies, the pulse repetition frequency (PRF) and wall filters should be set low enough to detect slow flow. When not adjusted properly, venous flow, especially reflux, can be missed. (For an overview of PRF and wall filters see Chapter 4. However, for an in-depth discussion on these items and implications on inaccurate use of these controls, we recommend a visit to www.pegasuslectures.com.) The best method is to have a set protocol working central to peripheral while scanning, doing a very repetitive set of steps at each location.

For evaluation of the deep veins the patient is typically in a supine position with a slight tilt (10–15°), with some variations as noted below.

Scanning the femoral vein

Follow along with the images in this section as the actual technique is described.

To begin scanning, apply a generous amount of gel to the anteromedial thigh from the groin to the knee. In a transverse view, start at the groin and locate the distal external iliac or common femoral artery and vein. This may be slightly above the inguinal crease. Perform a probe compression maneuver, making sure the vein walls fully coapt. This is best done with a slow deliberate movement. Next, move distally along the CFV until reaching

the split of the common femoral vein into the deep femoral (profunda femoris) and femoral vein. Perform a probe compression maneuver to assess the patency of the deep femoral and femoral veins. Follow the femoral vein distally, compressing every 1–2 cm along the entire length of the vein until you reach the adductor canal. At this point, it can be difficult to compress the femoral vein completely so it is best to assess the distal portion of the femoral vein using color flow imaging in a longitudinal view. Once passed the adductor canal, the femoral vein becomes the popliteal vein as it enters the popliteal space. This is discussed further below.

After completing the assessment of the deep veins in the thigh using probe compression, move centrally back to the groin and assess the deep veins using spectral Doppler. First, locate the common femoral artery and vein at the groin in a transverse view. Then rotate into a longitudinal view of the common femoral vein. At this point, evaluate the flow in the common femoral vein with spectral Doppler (Figure 5.9).

Assess for spontaneous and phasic flow (flow that stops during inspiration and returns during expiration), as well as augmentation with distal compression and with the Valsalva maneuver for possible reflux. Note that the Valsalva maneuver is an accurate test only to the first competent valve in the lower extremity. This is unfortunately not well understood by many and therefore Valsalva testing should be confined to the common femoral and saphenofemoral junction areas alone. Interpretation of the Doppler signals can be an art in itself. Augmentation for a patent vein should produce a clean crisp increase in flow. Any muted or blunted signal could indicate obstruction. Additionally, continuous flow may suggest thrombosis above the level under examination, and pulsatile flow could be indicative of cardiac overload issues. These phasic signals are best examined with the patient supine, or feet tilted down approximately 10–15°.

The common femoral vein should be examined in several locations. If possible, interrogation above the suprasaphenic valve and below the infrasaphenic valve should be performed. In this manner, any hemodynamic influence of the terminal valve of the saphenofemoral junction can be understood.

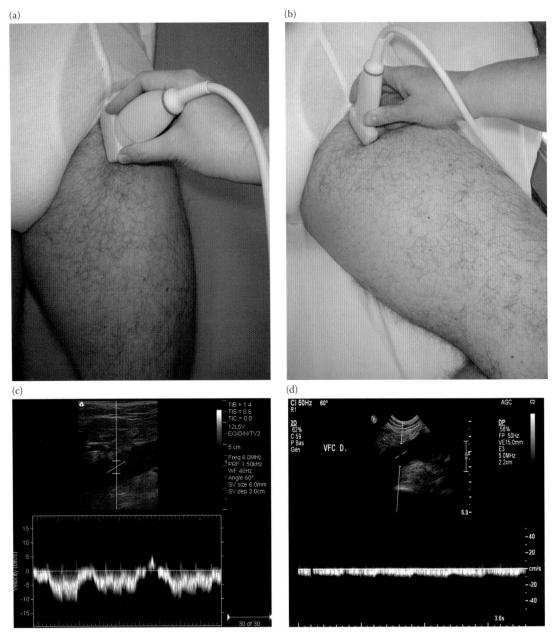

Figure 5.9 Probe in long axis on the CFV (a) standing or (b) supine; (c) phasicity of spectral wave form; (d) duplex showing loss of phasicity of CFV waveform.

Interrogation at the confluence of the femoral and profunda femoral vein is needed to document the status of the profunda femoris. Continue distally with spectral Doppler interrogation at the proximal femoral vein, mid-femoral vein, and distal femoral vein, and if possible the proximal popliteal vein, documenting these findings as per written protocols.

Scanning the popliteal vein

There are two methods for scanning the popliteal vein, either (1) reposition the patient by either having the patient rotate more onto the outer hip bending the knee slightly or into a lateral decubitus position with the knee bent slightly or (2) by approaching the patient from a posterior aspect.

Of note, the effect of popliteal compression with a hyperextended knee is something to be aware of, especially in the obese (Figure 5.10).[14, 15]

Begin just above the popliteal space and identify the popliteal artery and vein, remembering that the popliteal vein lies superficial to the artery with this approach. This is a key anatomic factor because in the thigh we typically use an anterior approach. However, when we scan from the posterior approach – that is to say from the popliteal fossa – the orientation of the vasculature is different. It is not that the vein and artery have changed position, but rather that the direction of insonation is different. From the posterior, the deep (popliteal) vein is closer to the skin level than the popliteal artery. Although this may seem different, it is only due to anatomic perspective being changed. Perform a probe compression maneuver, making sure the vein walls fully coapt. Next, move centrally along the popliteal vein to the adductor canal and visualize as much of the distal femoral

vein as possible. This is to ensure that a part of the distal femoral vein is not missed. Next, move distally, examining the popliteal vein with probe compressions about every 1–2 cm and following the popliteal vein to the posterior tibial and peroneal trunks. As performed previously, once compression maneuvers are completed, proceed with evaluating the flow along the popliteal vein using spectral (or color flow) Doppler. Assess for spontaneous and phasic flow, as well as augmentation with distal compression. Just like the common femoral vein at the saphenofemoral junction (SFJ), the popliteal vein should be examined above and below the SPJ. False retrograde flow in the popliteal vein may be seen at the SPJ level or higher in the presence of SPJ reflux, whereas retrograde flow distal to this level represents true deep venous reflux. Figure 5.10c visually demonstrates the 'siphon effect'. False deep vein reflux is often eliminated with removal of the varicose reservoir.[16, 17]

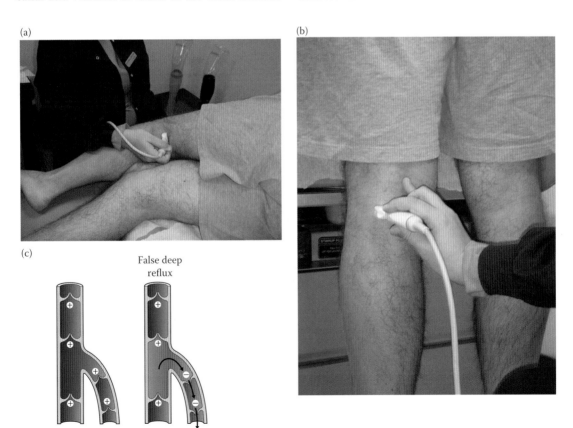

Figure 5.10 (a) Scanning the popliteal vein from a side approach, and (b) from a standing posterior approach. Panel (c) delineates a 'false' deep vein reflux due to siphon effect from the varicose reservoir.

Regarding unilateral evaluations of the deep veins of the thigh, for several reasons, but especially due to the 'art' of interpreting Doppler signals, it should be noted that a unilateral duplex evaluation for DVT should always include the evaluation of the contralateral common femoral vein. This is done for comparison reasons, as in many other areas of diagnostic procedures. Careful evaluation of the B-mode and especially of the spectral Doppler can help identify central issues relating to obstruction, extrinsic compression, or other pathologies. Evaluate Doppler signals for asymmetry, cardiovascular pulsatility, and respiratory phasicity. A recent case report from the *Journal of Vascular Ultrasound* supports this, stating 'findings on duplex ultrasound associated with pelvic venous obstruction are subtle, making obstruction more difficult to detect'.[7]

Scanning the deep calf veins

In many centers in the United States and around the world, routine scanning below the tibioperoneal junction is not performed. This decision should be made by the medical director of your laboratory and contained in the written protocols. ICAVL standards currently include calf veins for DVT studies; however, for insufficiency protocols the process of ruling out DVT in the calf is omitted. Of note, isolated anterior tibial vein thrombosis is limited to less than 2 percent of patients examined. As a result, when scanning calf veins, in the absence of thrombosis in the peroneal or posterior tibial veins, the anterior tibial veins are commonly not investigated.

When scanning the posterior tibial, anterior tibial, and peroneal veins, there are two basic approaches: (1) from the knee peripherally and (2) from the ankle centrally. One approach is not going to work every time, so it is best to be familiar with both approaches. Take advantage of venous hemodynamics, thus having the leg in a dependent position while the patient is sitting on the side of the examination table for calf vein interrogation can be extremely helpful (Figure 5.11a).

Remember that the calf veins are paired with their corresponding artery. Also bear in mind that blood flow is generally not spontaneous in the calf veins, therefore you must augment flow by distal compression. If you are having trouble locating the calf veins, color Doppler may be useful. In a transverse view, look for the artery flashing and then look for the

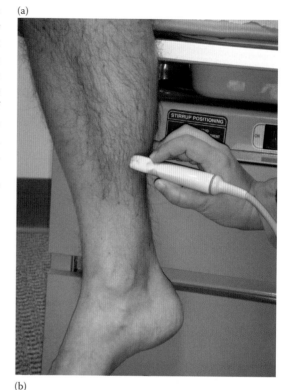

(a)

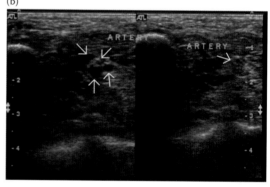

(b)

Figure 5.11 (a) Dependent position of leg for scanning of deep calf veins and (b) split screen image of posterior tibial vessels, with compression to the right.

corresponding veins. You can also try viewing the veins in a longitudinal axis using augmentation with distal compression to help locate the veins, again, using the flashing corresponding artery as a guide.

The posterior tibial veins lie posteromedial to the tibia and are best approached from the posteromedial aspect of the calf as noted in Figure 5.11a. At the ankle, the posterior tibial veins are located posterior to the medial malleolus where they are usually not too deep, and near the skin surface. Once located, perform probe compression maneuvers along the course of the posterior tibial veins to the common tibial trunk.

The anterior tibial veins are best visualized from an anterolateral approach (Figure 5.12). At the ankle, the anterior tibial veins are located just lateral to the tibia and course along the anterolateral aspect of the calf. At the knee, they dive under the fibula to join the popliteal vein. The most proximal portion of the anterior tibial veins must be visualized from a posterior approach since the tibia and fibula obstruct the view from the anterolateral approach. Again, perform probe compression maneuvers along the course of the anterior tibial veins to demonstrate compressibility and lack of thrombus.

The peroneal veins are best viewed at the same time as the posterior tibial veins, and can be visualized from the same posteromedial approach. A few centimeters above the ankle, you will see another set of paired veins with a corresponding artery that is in the far field of view. These are the peroneal veins. They lie just above the fibula, which shows as a bright, reflective surface on ultrasound. These can be followed centrally to the common peroneal trunk performing probe compressions every 2 cm (Figure 5.13).

The gastrocnemius veins, located in the calf, are typically described as dumb-bell shaped. One key factor regarding the gastrocnemius veins is to determine if the origin of these veins is the popliteal

(a)

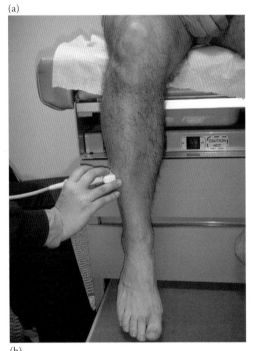

(b)

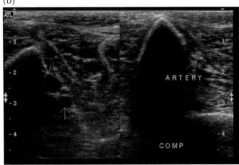

(a)

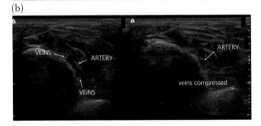

Figure 5.12 (a) Scanning of the anterior tibial veins using an anterior approach, and (b) spilt screen showing paired veins with artery on the left, and veins compressed on the right, leaving the artery visible.

Figure 5.13 (a) Scanning of the peroneal veins from the lateral approach, in the split screen duplex, the veins are indicated by arrows on the left, and compressed on the right, leaving only the artery visible.

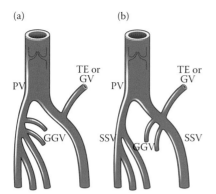

(a) (b)

TE or GV
PV
GGV SSV GGV SSV
TE or GV
PV

Figure 5.14 Variable location of the gastrocnemius vein connection to the popliteal or small saphenous vein.

vein or the small saphenous vein, as this may play into decision making if contemplating intervention on the small saphenous. Figure 5.14 describes these two anatomic presentations, but remember that in about 25 percent of cases a true SPJ does not exist.

At the end of this chapter (Figures 5.35 and 5.36), there are short form documents of this process. Also, in Chapter 6, sample written protocols are presented for DVT and reflux evaluations.

Author's commentary on deep system analysis

Unfortunately, focus on the superficial system, especially in those locations where a technologist or physician is new to phlebology and vascular ultrasound, evaluation of the deep venous system is minimized or completely overlooked. In limited numbers, authors in recent publications indicate this shortcoming; 'deep system interrogation was not routinely undertaken in this study.' One has to be fairly critical of these statements which may be mistaken, setting dubious precedent, by suggesting changing the standard of care. This is a definite error and great strides should be taken to reinstill the importance of deep system analysis. Comments overheard at some conferences have suggested a rationalization for this as 'the reimbursement code for a DVT study is the same one I use for a vein mapping (or reflux) study. I can't do twice the work for the same amount of reimbursement.' This clearly is a corruption of the ethical and moral duty to perform an adequate and complete study in clear contravention of a financial concept. The authors emphatically reject this approach. Deep system analysis is an important part of any venous

duplex, and the insinuation or belief that one can omit deep diagnosis completely for a reflux study is unconscionable.

As noted in the reflux protocol later in this chapter, evaluation of the deep veins including the popliteal and central (proximal) veins is critical for any phlebology patient. In advanced patients (C3–C6), a more detailed deep analysis and other modalities (air plethysmography) can also be very helpful.

As our understanding of the venous hemodynamics of the legs continues to develop, the omission of this deep system data prevents inquiring minds from understanding the relationship of superficial and deep system disease on global venous hemodynamics in the lower extremity. Published statements supporting the need to fully investigate the venous system include:

- Deep system reflux may not be a prerequisite for skin changes in patients with chronic venous insufficiency.[18]
- If peak velocity of reflux in the CFV is less than the peak velocity of reflux in the great saphenous vein (GSV), then stripping or ablation can eliminate the hydrostatic gradient and therefore deep system reflux is improved.[19]
- Kostas et al.[20] defined deep system reflux as the 'presence of reflux in any deep venous segment distal to the level of the common femoral vein and at least 1 cm away from the saphenofemoral or saphenopopliteal junctions where there was coexistent reflux at these sites'.
- Segmental deep system reflux at the saphenofemoral or saphenopopliteal junction is actually a steal or siphon effect due to the 'suction' created by the incompetent great or small saphenous vein.[21–23]
- Axial reflux in the superficial veins is poorly tolerated by the skin and subcutaneous tissues of the lower extremity and deserves surgical correction.[24]

The global nature of venous hemodynamics of the lower extremity is especially important in those patients in the C3–C6 range of the CEAP (clinical, etiologic, anatomic, pathophysiologic) class. Therefore, deep system investigation 'continues to be a fundamental part' of duplex examination for chronic venous disease. Deep system investigation for obstruction or insufficiency must not be minimized, omitted, or neglected for any patient seeking venous treatment,[25] especially those with advanced disease (C3–C6).

Scanning the iliac veins

For many reasons, phlebology and the related imaging of the venous system was historically focused on the infrainguinal region. Syndromes, such as the Nutcracker or May Thurner syndrome, although correctable through open repair, were not performed on a widespread basis. Endovenous techniques have evolved in recent years both from an imaging and a treatment approach standpoint, and there is growing interest on the suprainguinal venous structures. This section will provide an introduction to suprainguinal indications and techniques.

The indications for suprainguinal imaging should include symptoms and clinical presentation that would suggest central obstruction or occlusion. The most significant of these are compiled in Table 5.2. In any of these instances, it would be mandatory to investigate the iliac veins and inferior vena cava. Imaging with a curvilinear duplex probe

Table 5.2 Indications for suprainguinal venous duplex.

1. Pulmonary embolism, especially without any deep vein thrombosis (DVT) in the infrainguinal venous system
2. For any DVT in which the DVT extends above the inguinal ligament
3. Suspicion of compression of left iliac vein (May–Thurner syndrome)
4. Evaluation of outcomes of venous procedure (stenting, etc.)
5. Suspicion of ovarian vein issues

(typically 3 MHz) can be very helpful using proper techniques (Figure 5.15).

In Figures 5.16–5.18, the images below, the IVC and the iliac vein (and corresponding artery) are noted.

Imaging in this area can be more challenging due to respiratory movement, bowel gas and other factors. The typical venous evaluation is based on the ability

(a)

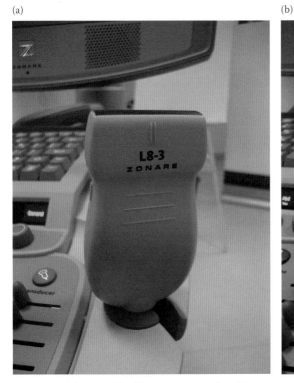

(b)

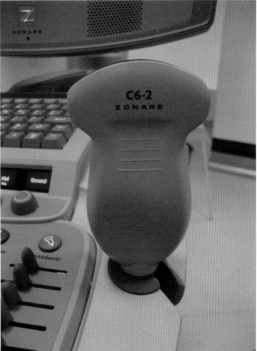

Figure 5.15 (a) A standard linear array probe; (b) the curved probe, which is used for iliac (and deeper) imaging.

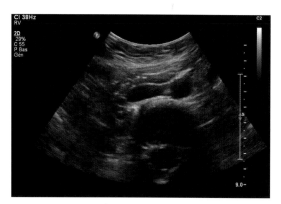

Figure 5.16 Inferior vena cava transverse view.

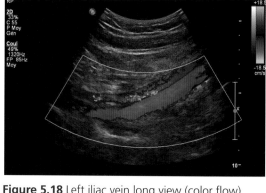

Figure 5.18 Left iliac vein long view (color flow).

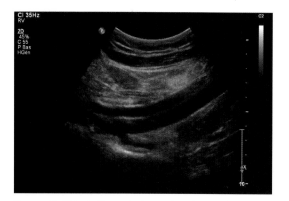

Figure 5.17 Left iliac vein long view (B-mode).

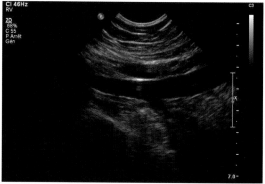

Figure 5.19 Right iliac vein prior to compression.

to perform a compression maneuver to demonstrate the lack of intraluminal thrombus. At times, this is able to be done as shown in Figures 5.19 and 5.20.

Although compression is the most reliable method, at times this is not achievable, at which time we rely on color flow imaging as in Figure 5.18. Note that the color scale is adjusted to 18.5 cm/s in this image, which provides information on both the arterial and venous flow. As true with all color Doppler, using the correct scale and PRF will allow for 'diagnostic' information to be gathered. Inappropriate settings will lead to inaccurate diagnosis (see Chapter 4 for more information on PRF).

Another key diagnostic tool is respiratory phasicity. In the Figure 5.21 note several points, the scale is set to 8.6 cm/s. Furthermore, we see the respiratory fluctuations on the left-hand side of the spectral tracing. Note, however, that with external compression on the abdomen, which is applied at about 2/3 s into the spectral wave form, there is a cessation of flow (i.e. spectral signal), and with

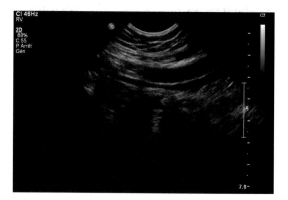

Figure 5.20 Right iliac vein with compression.

release, there is a sharp increase in venous flow with the initial return of blood flow.

As noted below in the description of the technique, each of these characteristics will be helpful to overcome the challenges and pitfalls that can occur in imaging this part of the body.

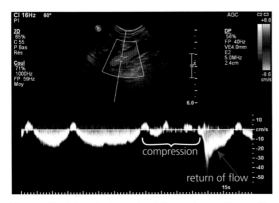

Figure 5.21 Respiratory phasicity and cessation with abdominal compression.

Technique for suprainguinal imaging

The patient is typically placed in a supine position with slight elevation of the head (~10°). Start determining the flow in the common femoral veins (flux) to check for iliocaval patency. This is done with observation of the phasicity of flow with augmentation with the thigh compression maneuver. As noted elsewhere, changes can be suggestive of central obstruction, however the absence of change is *non-diagnostic*. In the most basic method, begin by identification of the common femoral vein in a transverse view, and scan central to this following the vein to the confluence of the iliac veins, and continue proximal to examine the vena cava. By performing this examination 'in continuity', several pitfalls can be avoided.

Alternatively, some experts in the field suggest beginning in the abdomen and finding the psoas muscle. This muscle is readily seen through the abdomen, and the iliac vein sits on top of the muscle, so by finding the psoas as a landmark and fanning the probe laterally the iliac vein will come into view.

Pitfalls include the confusion of a very large ovarian vein with the iliac – note that the ovarian vein is more lateral that the iliac. It depends on the level; the ovarian vein crosses the iliac vein forward and then goes lateral to join the renal vein (left) or the IVC (right), but this is a relatively less common mistake. Also this could occur using B-mode with a dilated ureter, however with Doppler interrogation this mistake could be avoided. For these reasons, we believe the best method is simply to find the common femoral vein (a known landmark) and trace it proximal.

In a normal situation, a smooth compression on the abdomen will produce a cessation of flow in the area due to the increased central pressure. Upon release, there will initially be a surge or increased flow due to the backed up flow from the legs, which will quickly return to a normal baseline level. In case of thrombosis, venous flow signals may show decreased phasicity, low but continuous flow. Ultimately, the examination is sensitive, especially with comparison of contralateral sides for variances.

Today, we have efficient probe design, typically a convex probe with variable imaging frequencies of 2–5 MHz for iliac imaging. Harmonic imaging, which increases contrast, is extremely helpful for accurate imaging of these veins. Due to the deeper location, as compared to the vascular flow in the lower extremities, working knowledge of the duplex 'knobology' will help assure accurate diagnostic techniques.

As noted above, and this is worth repeating, the sequence of events in evaluation of the iliac area are:

- First step: direct B-mode imaging and testing for direct visualization of intraluminal thrombus. If the thrombus is slightly more echogenic, which happens as the thrombus ages, we can see the clot itself. If the thrombus is fresh (or acute) B-mode may not be diagnostic on its own.
- Second step: although this can be limited due to body habitus, external compressions are sometimes possible in this area (similar to what is done below the inguinal ligament). In addition, we can use compressions applied to the thigh to provide increased flow for evaluation as we examine these vessels either with spectral or color Doppler.
- Third step: use of color imaging is extremely helpful in looking for vein filling without deficits (incomplete filling). As noted above, to achieve good filling, compression of the thigh (squeeze for distal augmentation), is often required. This can be achieved using hand compressions. Again to emphasize the point, adjust to low PRF, and color gains, etc., for this

area, so that the examination is as diagnostic as possible.

As noted in the figures above, and some of the images below, very good views of the vessels can be achieved in long axis using the color flow imaging. Also, during this portion, the confluence of the internal iliac vein can also be clearly seen for additional diagnostic information regarding direction of flow, as noted below in which we see the left iliac vein with reversal of flow (Figure 5.22). This is due to May Thurner syndrome.

The approach above is primarily based on an anterior-type approach. In some cases, these views will be limited. A secondary and more lateral approach can be taken to complement the process, and adapting to each situation based on patient anatomy is the key.

The pitfalls that can be encountered are a little more challenging in this part of the body as compared to the infrainguinal vasculature. One of the most common pitfalls is the presence of bowel gas.

If you encounter bowel gas, there are a few techniques that are helpful. First, change angle and approach. Next, using the probe, you are sometimes able to 'milk' the gas along the bowel and create an open window through which to image. Another option is to ask the patient to relax the abdominal wall as they have a tendency to tense up while imaging, so a relaxed patient with soft (relaxed) abdomen is key. Ask the patient to take a deep inspiration as if for moving the bowels, which may result in a better view. The other factor is 'time', as bowel movement is

a constant bodily function, sometimes it is convenient to scan the contralateral side and return later during the examination to the spot which was proving difficult. Interestingly, body habitus can be a problem, and contrary to popular belief, a thinner person may prove more difficult with bowel gas than a heavier one. For larger patients, the anterior approach is more difficult and a lateral approach is much easier. Although not really a body habitus issue, pregnancy also provides a challenge with the anterior approach. In this situation, it is common to only have an adequate viewing window (access) using the lateral approach.

Other pitfalls include things like: the postoperative condition of the patient and previous or concurrent scarring. Immediately postoperatively, pain and dressing issues, including drainage, can be a challenge. If surgery was very recent, it is a good idea to use a sterile technique (including sterile gel) to avoid contamination of the open wound. At times, this may prove too cumbersome or nondiagnostic, and if so, changing to another imaging modality, such as computed tomography venography (CTV), may be required.

There are many conditions that can be seen, and with good technique can be seen well, with regard to the iliac venous structures. Some of the conditions that can be diagnosed include, but are not limited to, the following: normal and abnormal anatomic variations, such as duplication of the IVC, atresia of IVC, aneurysm of IVC, which is quite atypical, and external compression with conditions such as pelvic masses, i.e. carcinoma. Other items that can be appreciated include follow up for IVC filters, often the filter due to its high echogenicity can be located above or below the renals, to determine filter migration, if it is tilted, etc. Evaluation of the renal veins is also accomplished and if there is DVT in the IVC, determination of the central end of the DVT can be achieved. Typically for evaluation of the IVC, approaches can include anterior, right anterior lateral, right lateral and, at times, a transcostal view or retroperitoneal view of the IVC may be possible.

Below are a series of images and descriptions of findings using suprainguinal imaging.

Nutcracker syndrome is more challenging with ultrasound (Figure 5.23), and there is an absence of good criteria for its evaluation. One concept

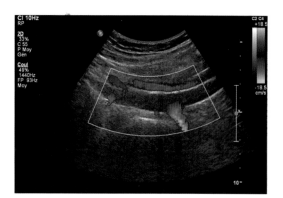

Figure 5.22 Reversal of flow in the left internal iliac vein.

involved thinking of the variation in compression between the standing and supine positions. Evaluation with IVC is helpful with intravascular ultrasound (IVUS), but it is both invasive and expensive. Olivier Pichot, MD indicates that typically this is best evaluated with phlebography in France. In addition, the termination of the left iliac vein is difficult to see in many patients due to imaging difficulties, and therefore suspicion can be high.

Acute DVT as noted in Figure 5.24, and its sequelae can be seen with duplex in this area. Other related applications would include serial investigation of DVT for remnants or recanalizations, including the development of lumbar or palmar collaterals.

As noted in Figure 5.25, duplex can be very helpful in the evaluation of the development of intimal hyperplasia. As such, applications like post-procedure examination for angioplasty and stent placement, and vein patency following an intervention can be performed.

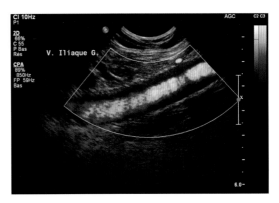

Figure 5.25 Intimal hyperplasia post-stenting.

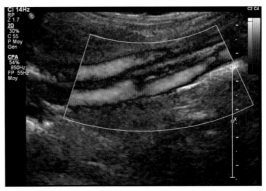

Figure 5.26 Fibrosis sequelae post-thrombotic event.

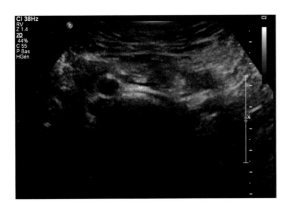

Figure 5.23 Inferior vena cava compression.

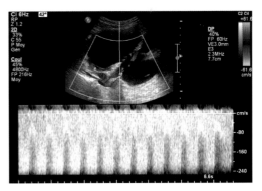

Figure 5.27 External iliac compression by seroma and below, the corresponding increased spectral flow.

Other changes in the vein wall can be noted on duplex. Chronic conditions including scarring/fibrosis, recanalization, intraluminal webs, hypotrophic size changes can be observed (Figure 5.26).

Other external compression pathologies can also be noted as in Figure 5.27, including the increased flow velocities noted from color changes at the compression area.

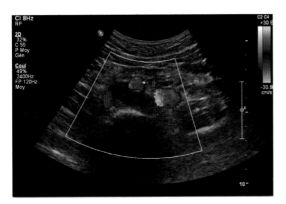

Figure 5.24 Deep vein thrombosis.

Perforating vein scanning

Duplex scanning of perforating veins can be broken down into basic concepts which help with understanding of the process. As described in the anatomy section, a perforator by definition 'perforates' the deep fascia. In the lower leg, the paratibial perforators connect the great saphenous vein with the deep system, however the posterior tibial perforators are typically connected to the posterior accessory saphenous vein of the leg (previously the posterior arch vein), and the deep system (not the GSV). It is also helpful to think that perforators are either exit (leak points) or re-entry perforators, the latter in which venous volume re-enters the deep compartment. The number of perforators in the leg has been noted to be 100–200, although most are quite small. Those of interest in duplex examinations are typically larger and more easily seen.

Probe orientation is also a key consideration when scanning perforators. Typically, we think of the probe as being either vertically or horizontally oriented in order to acquire good transverse or long axis images. Perforator anatomy is more variable and meanders through the body. Due to this, once a perforator is localized, the probe should be slowly rotated and adjusted to obtain the best possible image of the course of the perforator. This often results in odd probe orientation angles in order to get optimal imaging results (Figure 5.28).

There are two approaches to perforator imaging that are most effective, (1) fascial examination and (2) sourcing of varicose blood flow.

With fascial examination, the key is to identify the deep fascial boundary and to scan methodically with focus on the fascia, looking for 'breaks' which appear as shadows across the hyperechoic fascial boundary. Typically, scanning is done with a slightly faster than normal speed, seeking the break, and then focusing in on that location once a break is noticed. In scanning for the posterior tibial perforators, begin with the probe located posterior and above the posterior tibial veins, scan upward along the calf. At the top of the calf, move the probe one probe length anterior, and descend along the leg towards the ankle. In using this approach, a scan zone equal to the width of the probe is sequentially performed from posterior

(a)

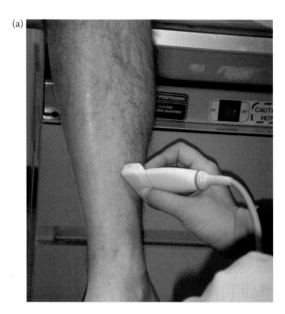

(b)

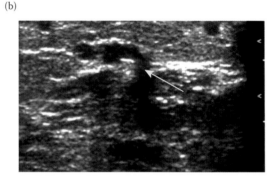

Figure 5.28 (a) Variable probe orientation for perforator imaging (not the typical horizontal or vertical approach) and (b) the corresponding duplex image of the perforator. The 'fascial break' is noted with an arrow.

to anterior, focusing on the fascial boundary, seeking the breaks indicative of perforator location.

'Sourcing' varicose flow perforator identification is another technique for perforator localization. In this method, a varicosity is imaged and traced (or sourced using the swinging column of blood technique described by Obermeyer and Garzon[26]) along its course. The concept in this approach is to follow the varix until the observation of a vein diving deeper towards and perforating the fascia is noted. This can be more challenging in that with superficial varicosities, the slightest increase in probe pressure will shrink the size of the perforator suggesting its termination at the skin level and not through a terminal perforator. One clue for finding terminal perforators is that typically the varicosity will dilate near the connection to the perforator due to transmitted pressure. Therefore, closer examination is suggested at points where the varix increases in size.

With either approach, localization of clinically significant perforators needs to be accomplished in conjunction with the patient's presenting varicose configuration, the patient's symptoms (pain), and ultimately (in addition to a normal or standard saphenous protocol) if the source of the varicose pathology has not already been identified. Often perforator dilation is related to the venous hypertension of the superficial network. *Once the venous hypertension is removed with intervention, the size and function of the perforators need to be redetermined, as some re-entry or terminal perforators return to normal size and function once a grossly incompetent saphenous trunk is ablated.*[27] Recently, Gloviczki et al.[28] defined a 'pathologic' perforator as one that is greater than 3.5 mm, with bidirectional or outward flow, and adjacent to an ulcer.

Examination techniques for superficial system scanning

Prior to scanning the superficial system, it is often best to understand the prevalence of patterns and distribution of the reflux typically encountered. Table 5.3 describes the prevalence of these distribution patterns. Note there is a 9 percent incidence of non-saphenous reflux patterns, in which case no reflux will be noted in the GSV or small saphenous vein (SSV) and investigation needs to be pushed further for diagnosis and clinical correlation.

A description of the general approach to superficial scanning will be delineated next, followed by key concepts regarding reflux and interpretation of studies. Figures will illustrate the process described.

Scanning the superficial system requires an investigator who is interested in the outcome of the examination. Rather, someone who will compare the test results with the clinical picture to see if they match up, and if not, will keep going to find the source of the problem. One example of how this does not happen is the sonographer who scans the leg according to a known protocol, generates a

Table 5.3 Prevalence of reflux in saphenous networks.

Location	No.	%
GSV	111	65
SSV	33	19
GSV + SSV	12	7
Non-saphenous	15	9
Total	171	100

GSV, great saphenous vein; SSV, small saphenous vein. Data from Labropoulos N, Tiongson J, Pryor L et al. Nonsaphenous superficial vein reflux. *Journal of Vascular Surgery* 2001; **34**: 872–7.

report that indicates the lack of reflux in the GSV and SSV, even though there are gross varicosities along the anterior lateral thigh, descending along the lateral thigh and leg. In this case, a true investigator would go beyond the protocol and find the refluxing non-saphenous source that leads to the varicose complex. In order to avoid this type of mistake, it is always a good idea to examine the patient with a 'focused' visual inspection and query them about their problem prior to beginning the scan. In this way, a sonographer can seek out the source of the problem during the normal protocols. If the source is identified, no other information needs to be gathered. However if not, additional information is required until sufficient data are provided for accurate diagnosis. As noted in the Society of Vascular Ultrasound's performance guidelines,[10] excerpts below:

2.1 Obtain a complete, pertinent history by interview of the patient or patient's representative and review of the patient's medical record. A pertinent history includes:
a. *Relevant risk factors for lower extremity venous insufficiency, previous deep vein and/or superficial vein thrombosis (DVT/SVT), lower extremity trauma, history of venous ulcers and/or varicosities, familial history of varicose veins.*
b. *Current medications or therapies.*
c. *Results of other relevant diagnostic procedures.*

2.2 Complete a limited or focused physical examination, which includes observation and localization of the presence of any signs or symptoms of peripheral venous disease: swelling, pain, tenderness, discoloration, varicosities, and ulceration.

3a 'sonographic findings are analyzed throughout the course of the examination to ensure that sufficient data are provided to the physician to direct patient management and render a final diagnosis record.'

Patient assessment

As noted above, obtain a patient history and perform a limited physical examination which includes looking for any signs or symptoms of peripheral venous disease, such as swelling, pain, tenderness, palpable cord, discoloration, varicosities, and ulceration. This should be done with the patient standing in a well-lit area. The purpose of this is to focus on the patient's complaints so that you are able to determine if the findings match the clinical condition of the patient.

Patient positioning

When scanning the superficial system of the lower extremities, patient positioning is vital for this examination to be of value. Venous reflux is a disease that is gravity dependent. Therefore, if at all possible, examinations should be undertaken with the patient in the **standing position**.[29] If this is not a realistic option, a steep tilt table may be an option. When scanning the calf or SSV, a seated position with the leg dangling over the side of the examination table can also be used. Any determinations of reflux done in the supine position will have higher false-negative values,[30,31] and therefore should be avoided. Additionally, vein size measurements will not be accurate if measured in the supine position, as the hydrostatic effect on vein diameter is removed.[32] This will be discussed further below.

Equipment and probe selection

A high-resolution ultrasound machine with real-time imaging, superior gray scale, an integrated pulsed, range-gated Doppler is required. Record keeping and storage is critical, therefore the ability to record the Doppler waveform and image is highly recommended. Most current ultrasound systems available today provide for video output in digital format which, along with most other medical records is becoming the preferred format. At the end of a given study, a series of image prints or video clips should be stored for the interpreting physician to review and dictate the report. Also, these digital prints need to be archived properly according to state or local laws for medical record storage.

A linear array transducer with a range of 7.5–12 MHz is typically available and should be used for evaluating the superficial venous system.

Superficial scanning is best done using as many of the ultrasonic landmarks as possible to facilitate proper vessel identification and understanding of the pathology encountered. In each scenario described below, place warm gel on the leg, and take a prescan of the leg to help identify structures prior to image acquisition and labeling to prevent identification mistakes from taking place.

Calf and small saphenous vein

Begin scanning the calf at the mid-calf level and find the small saphenous within the saphenous compartment (Figure 5.29). Perform a prescan in the transverse approach by scanning at a moderate pace up and down the calf and posterior thigh. At this point, we are casually observing any large or dilated branches or perforators and getting a general orientation for the anatomy of the small saphenous and the thigh extension. Of particular note during this phase, the fascia compartment at the mid-calf is fairly thick with space on each side of the SSV. Moving up the calf towards the popliteal fossa, this compartment narrows, and in most instances will thin out so much that the only item in the compartment will be the SSV without any other space (Figure 5.30). By scanning in the transverse, information related to perforators, large branches and intersaphenous connections will be able to be observed and noted. As a general rule, any tributary that is 50 percent or larger as compared to the saphenous vein typically needs to be mapped out (50 percent rule). Branches or tributaries less than 50 percent of the saphenous size are typically less important, and this rule of thumb helps to eliminate the need to trace out every single branch to its termination.

(a)

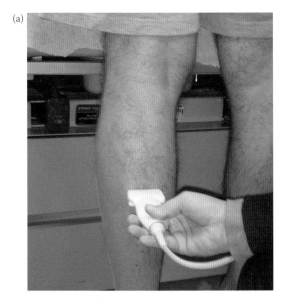

it is the intersaphenous vein commonly called the Giacomini vein.

There are two main patterns of SSV reflux to be aware of: (1) primary SSV incompetence and (2) SSV incompetence distal to an intersaphenous branch (Figure 5.31).

As noted by Obermeyer and Garzon,[26] crossover patterns from one saphenous system to the other exist in a fair number of cases (21 percent) and need to be understood for properly directed treatment. This is typically a good stopping point to make a few notes on the technical worksheet and create the vein map of the SSV distribution.

(a)

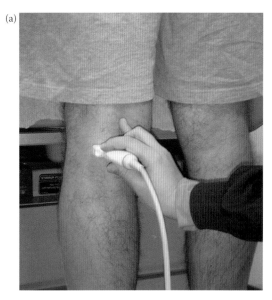

(b)

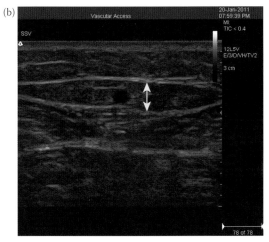

Figure 5.29 (a,b) Small saphenous vein at mid-calf, note the wider fascial compartment (indicated by arrows) making vessel identification easier.

Once parameters have been established, you are ready to start documenting information. Typically for the SSV, diameter and reflux determinations are made 3 cm below the SPJ and a mid-calf measurement should also be made.[8] Also, a determination will be made for the cranial extension (if present) as it ascends the posterior thigh. If the cranial extension is present, trace this vein central to see if it becomes the infragluteal vein, and dives deep to connect to the profunda femoris vein. If it courses medially to join the posterior accessory of the GSV,

(b)

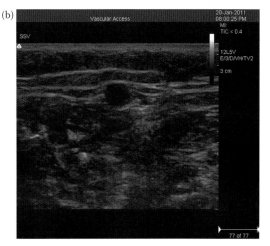

Figure 5.30 (a,b) Small saphenous vein at proximal calf with very thin compartment noted.

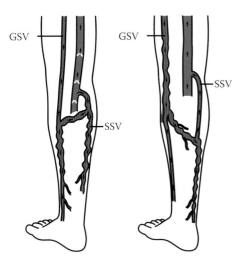

Figure 5.31 Small saphenous vein reflux patterns. On the left is primary incompetence of the SSV and on the right is a crossover pattern from GSV incompetence.

Next, ask the patient to turn around to face the sonographer. The patient should be standing with the leg to be examined externally rotated and their weight on the contralateral leg. Be sure that the heel is flat on the floor, otherwise, a mild, but persistent systolic contraction of the calf occurs when the heel is elevated that can affect results (Figure 5.32).

Scanning the GSV is all about the fascial compartment (or canal). Begin at mid-thigh and with an adequate amount of gel, prescan up and down the thigh to get a general idea of the path of the GSV and any large tributaries or other findings. At the junction, an anterior accessory saphenous, posterior accessory saphenous, or other veins can be present which could make correct identification of the GSV at the junction slightly more difficult (if you were to start scanning at the level of the common femoral vein). By starting in the compartment at the mid-thigh and tracing the vein proximal, proper identification of the GSV is easily accomplished.

One of the most important clues to reflux patterns will be the size or diameter of the saphenous vein in its compartment (Figure 5.33). The saphenous vein will typically be smaller below a tributary where reflux leaves the saphenous compartment. This 'change in size' is a key clue to tracing out reflux.

Keeping this in mind, we are ready to scan the GSV and gather information about flow dynamics

in the thigh. Typically, three determinations of reflux are initially made for the GSV, one near the junction, one at mid-thigh, and one at the knee. If all three agree, then we assume that the flow is the same at all three levels. If, however, two are different, additional determinations are required

(a)

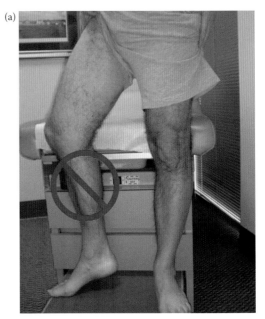

(b)

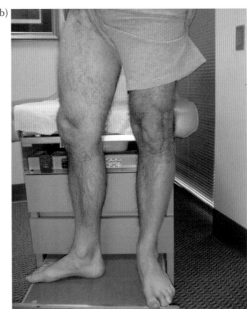

Figure 5.32 Positioning of the patient for GSV examination (a) with an inappropriate calf systole and (b) correct positioning.

(a)

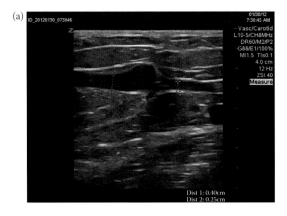

(b)

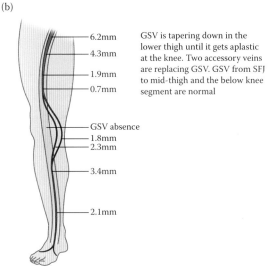

6.2mm
4.3mm
1.9mm
0.7mm

GSV is tapering down in the lower thigh until it gets aplastic at the knee. Two accessory veins are replacing GSV. GSV from SFJ to mid-thigh and the below knee segment are normal

GSV absence
1.8mm
2.3mm

3.4mm

2.1mm

Figure 5.33 Change in size of the great saphenous vein. (a) The reduction in size of the GSV from the left to the right side of this image is suggestive of reflux leaving the saphenous canal via a tributary. (b) Change in size of the saphenous vein along its course (courtsey N Labropolous).

in the area between the two differing points. By segmenting the GSV in this manner, we can evaluate the flow along its course investigating further where flow changes occur. Others 'recommend to test the saphenous veins every 3–5 cm for compressibility and reflux'.

Using the transverse approach (and size as a general guide), scan out the course of the GSV from the groin to the knee. Again, this is best accomplished by finding the GSV at mid-thigh in the fascia and tracing it up to the junction. Diameter measurements are best made in the transverse or short axis approach (to include the vein wall[8]) and therefore

the anteroposterior diameter should be measured. Document the size on the GSV near the junction, at the mid-thigh and additionally at the knee. While gathering this information, make a mental note of the anterior accessory saphenous vein or the posterior accessory saphenous vein, if noticed, as well as any large tributaries coming off the GSV along the thigh. After the diameter is gathered, go back and perform spectral analysis at each of these three levels using a calf compression/release maneuver. Reflux is measured during muscular diastole, or after 'release' of the distal calf compression. Spectral analysis should be taken in the long axis with the gate open over the entire vein (wall to wall) and using an appropriate angle of 45–60° is optimal. After these determinations are made, additional measurements should be taken to establish the size and, if reflux is present, in either of the posterior or anterior accessory saphenous veins. At this point, we are focusing only on the veins in the saphenous compartment. Once all these measurements and reflux determinations are complete, we can investigate from the saphenous compartment up to the skin level, checking and tracing out any large tributaries noted (again using the *50 percent rule* as described earlier for the SSV, and not tracing out smaller insignificant tributaries). By focusing on the saphenous compartment first, we typically find the 'source' of the flow that feeds into the more superficial varicosities. This also simplifies our process to what is most important first. Similarly, Labropolous *et al.*[32] comment on saphenous vein measurements that truly reflect the size of the vein, stating that measurements should be taken in non-aneurysmal locations. Furthermore, focal dilations were more prevalent in GSVs than in 'true' varicosities, or put another way, 98 percent of varicosities occur in tributaries and not the actual truncal GSV. They further defined that 'any vein outside the fascia was considered an accessory or tributary (even if it left the fascia and then re-entered).'

This is typically a good point to stop, make notes, and create the vein map of the thigh section of the leg on the technical worksheet.

Now that the thigh is done, we need to focus on the GSV in the (lower) leg. In the proximal part of the lower leg, the saphenous vein can again be sometimes difficult to correctly identify, there is often hypo- or aplasia of the GSV at or below the knee (Figure 5.33b).

The most useful method is to find the GSV at the ankle along the medial malleolus. By finding the vein at this level, it is again in the saphenous compartment (although thinned out) and we can trace it more central towards the knee and the segment previously scanned. The GSV is located along the medial posterior ridge of the tibia as it ascends in the lower leg until just below the knee where it curves posterior. In the lower leg, diagnostic information is typically gathered for the GSV in two locations, one at the proximal calf and one slightly below half way to the ankle. At each of these levels, a diameter is measured and then reflux determination is made. Of particular note is the posterior accessory great saphenous vein (PAGSV) of the leg, previously called either the posterior arch vein or the vein of Leonardo. The lower section of the leg is where we see the greatest number of perforating veins. The posterior tibial perforating veins (old Cockett's perforators) connect the posterior accessory saphenous vein of the leg to the posterior tibial veins. They typically do not connect to the distal great saphenous vein itself. Varicosities along this section of the leg are typically prevalent, so scan initially over the GSV itself, focusing on the compartment, as noted above. Once the course of the GSV is understood, go back and trace out the varices to their origins.

In summary, we have scanned the SSV, the GSV in the thigh, the anterior accessory great saphenous vein (AAGSV), and PAGSV if present, and then, the distal GSV, stopping between each step to create a vein map of our findings. If there are any veins or varices which are not yet understood, additional steps to 'source' these veins need to be carried out. This is done by placing the ultrasound probe over any remaining veins, and using light probe pressure, tracing these in a detailed fashion to determine the source. At several points along the way, check for reflux to ensure proper understanding of the course of the vein. Also, while this description lists several recommended locations for determination of caliber and reflux, additional points may be required based on the individual anatomic pathology of each patient.

Note that at the end of this chapter a short bullet point document is provided which can serve as a guide for the beginner in this process. Forms and worksheets are provided in Chapter 6 which is dedicated to protocols, documentation, and samples.

Reflux examination considerations and variability in reflux curves

It is generally understood that approximately 10 percent of the blood volume is contained in the superficial venous system of the lower extremities.[33] With increasing age, there is an increasing prevalence of reflux disease.[34] Although the exact biologic or developmental causes of venous insufficiency are not known, some patterns have become apparent; in the majority of those with superficial functional impairment, the great saphenous vein is involved, and to a much lesser extent the small saphenous vein.[35]

We do understand that reflux is due to hydrostatic pressure gradients which occur during diastole in the lower extremity, and because of the anatomic structure of the leg, reflux is typically associated with a change in compartment.[36] Additionally, published information indicates that the condition of the venous system, especially with regard to reflux and chronic venous disease, like other disease processes, is not static. The extent of reflux and its specific patterns change with or without changes in the associated symptoms in some cases. For this reason, a repeat examination should be performed to monitor changes in size, extent and distribution of retrograde flow and other pathologic measures[37] at about six month intervals.

Particular consideration needs to be paid to the changing thought regarding the *origin of reflux*. Historically, the belief was that reflux originated proximally resulting in a descending or waterfall concept. More recently, Pittaluga, Bernardini and Labropolous have noted that reflux develops distally and superficially, probably due to the lack of support in the epifascial space, progressing from trbutaries to the saphenous trunk, then ascending to eventually lead to sapheno-femoral junctional incompetence. This represents the ascending theory. And therefore, reflux can start in the epifascial space or saphenous compartment, and progresses proximal or distal over years." [37, 38, 39]

Definition

Labropolous and others defined the determination of reflux based on valve closure times and abnormal retrograde flow.[40] The values currently accepted for pathologic reflux are: greater than 1.0 second in

Table 5.4 Definition of reflux.[a]

Region	Pathologic reflux (s)
Femoropopliteal	>1
Superficial	>0.5
Perforator	>0.35

[a] A new definition was set out in the American Venous Forum/Society for Vascular Surgery guidelines for 'pathologic' perforators as those 'perforating veins with outward flow ≥500 ms duration, vein diameter ≥3.5 mm, and located underneath healed or active ulcers (CEAP class C5–C6)'.[28]

the femoropopliteal (deep) veins, greater than 0.5 seconds in the saphenous systems, and greater than 0.35 seconds for perforating veins, as noted in Table 5.4. As noted earlier, duration of reflux is the key consideration. **Spectral analysis is like time delay photography in that the curve shows a temporal window extending for several seconds. Static color flow images are not adequate to document reflux, as they depict only one instant in time, and do not allow for quantization of the reflux.**

Position

Gravity dependence on determination of reflux during duplex studies is well known. Although there are various approaches describing tilt tables, a standing examination of the vein system of the lower extremities has become the standard of care.[30, 31, 34, 41–46] Therefore, unless impractical, an examination should be performed in the standing position, testing the non-weight-bearing leg.[47] This latter aspect to avoid muscular systole in the leg muscles is addressed further below. Insonation of the great saphenous system is best performed using an anterior approach with the leg externally rotated. The small saphenous, popliteal fossa, and posterior aspect of the leg is best approached from behind, with the knee slightly bent forward. Although there is some resistance from technologists to ergonomically adapt to this position, it is relatively easy and practical to attain in most settings. One author suggested having the patients stand for 10 full minutes prior to determining venous cross-sectional area[48] and this seems excessive. Meissner *et al.*[49] describe active dorsiflexion causing reduction in ambulatory venous pressure studies, i.e. hydrostatic

pressure in the standing patient. Furthermore, they report that hydrostatic pressure is restored after 31 seconds of resuming a static standing position.[49] In daily practice, this author uses about 2 minutes of standing position, during which a brief physical inspection of the legs is performed. This not only allows for a directed duplex having performed the physical examination, but also venous system 'equilibration' with the patient in the standing position prior to starting a duplex.

Time of day

Although the position for reflux determination has a relative consensus, the time of day to perform a study is a variable for debate because of its effects on the results of reflux. In most cases, the time of day a duplex is performed has little impact. However, in roughly 30 percent of patients, differential results may be obtained. Some argue that a morning examination is more accurate, while others seem to prefer an afternoon examination.[49, 50] A recent multicenter trial (the INVEST study) described the difficulties in reproducibility and repeatability of duplex studies, which described how these figures improved with training and use of a standardized protocol.[51] In agreement, as noted by Gibson's group, things like 'GSV diameter measured by duplex scanning, can have interobserver and intraobserver variability depending on time of day'.[52] The INVEST study indicated that the most repeatable studies were performed in the morning, with the patient standing. Although standing is something we agree with, we believe that the so-called 'errors' that were increased in afternoon studies were actually that sensitivity became an issue as most understand that reflux can be 'worse' in the afternoon in borderline patients (typically C2), so once again, clinical correlation becomes even more important. By taking a good clinical history, the patient's lifestyle can be better understood. For instance, a person who works third shift (overnight), and presents to the laboratory for a diagnostic study in the early morning should be considered the same as a person who works during the day and presents to the office in the late afternoon; the concept being they have been standing/working for many hours prior to their examination. Due to this lifestyle distinction, this subgroup was eliminated from statistical analysis in one published study.[43] In afternoon examinations, as would be expected, increased incidence of swelling and reflux, which are more prevalent in perforating veins, was noted. This variable has been controlled for in some studies using air plethysmography and photoplethysmography techniques. Although the time of day variable is recognized, it may prove impractical for patient scheduling. It needs to be taken into account when results either do not correlate with symptoms, or appear contrary to physical findings, i.e. false negatives. The authors of the INVEST study strongly suggest reporting the time of day a study was performed in the final interpretation and dictated report.

Reflux curves

Many authors have attempted to understand retrograde flow and reflux curves. Attempts at quantification have varied from: simple time scales, volume measurements based on vein caliber, flow rate, and estimation formulas,[53] to determination of area under the spectral curves and more complex ratio-type analysis relating the area of forward flow compared to area of reversed flow on the spectral wave form.[54, 55] Debate regarding the severity of a high velocity – short duration reflux wave versus a low but sustained reflux wave abound, but without real consensus (Figure 5.34). As described by Labropoulos et al.,[40] 'when a large incompetent vein empties into a small capacitor, peak vein velocity is high, but duration is short. When the refluxing vein is small and the capacitor is large, velocity is low and RF duration is long … and no definite conclusions can be made.' The size and shape of the varicose network, more specifically the capacitor into which the reflux flows is a large factor on these issues. A larger diameter straight vein will produce a stronger effect on a smaller distal region than a varicose complex with many vessels and significant curvilinear distributions. Our duplex determinations measure reflux time, the surrogate marker of valve closure time. Thus, any attempt to quantify reflux is a practical impossibility due to all the factors: venous tone, distensibility, temperature, hydration, time of day, length of time standing, repeated attempts at augmentation, hormonal influences (monthly fluctuations or in those who are pregnant), cardiac load, and respiratory cycles to name a few, which can

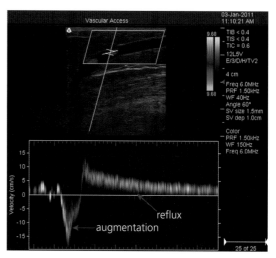

Figure 5.34 Demonstration of a good crisp augmentation and reflux.

affect the spectral curve from which interpretations are based. We strive to analyze results, knowing that control of these variables is impractical, at least at the current time.

Augmentation concepts

Most clinicians know and understand the calf muscle pump. There are, however, several muscle 'pumps' in the leg contributing to venous flow. From a practical perspective, there are several methods to mimic the effect of calf muscle pump diastole, and thus elicit retrograde flow. For research and publication applications, many believe that the use of cuffs with large bore rapid deflation abilities inflated to specific values of cuff pressures allows for reproducibility.[38] Several clinicians within phlebology settings are moving towards this format. In everyday situations, several less cumbersome techniques seem to be more commonly employed and will be discussed below.

1. Distal or calf augmentation. Manual hand compressions should be either over the calf muscle, or directly over the varicose capacitance bed which is connected to the vein being tested. The difficulty here is the variability of the force of the compression, which can include the size of the sonographer's hand, but is hard to reproduce from one person to the next. When

performing a compression, it is best to squeeze, and pause (or hold) for about 0.25 s, and then release. This allows for precise interpretation of the two phases (systole and diastole). Furthermore, it allows for the spectral curve to display the change in direction of flow between the two phases (see Figure 5.34).

2. Valsalva. Produces higher intra-abdominal pressures, typically done with forceful contraction of the abdomen. This technique is excellent for evaluation of the terminal and subterminal valves at the saphenous junction. It requires understanding that flow from the superior tributary veins of the saphenofemoral junction have descending flow, i.e. draining the abdominal wall through the SFJ. The differentiation of terminal and subterminal valve incompetence has been effectively done using this technique. This technique can be more challenging to the novice, but adds information about the saphenous arch. A standardized approach to Valsalva was recently described using a pressure blow tube by De Maeseneer *et al.* in the UIP consensus document.[8] Although this helps to standardize the pressure exerted during Valsalva, widespread routine adoption of this method is unlikely. Malgor and Labropolous state that 'valsalva manoeuver is used only when there is no reflux with the compression/release test'[29]

3. Active dorsiflexion and plantar flexion. Technically more difficult for the ultrasound examiner due to patient movement, pulsed Doppler aiming, and patient compliance. However, active muscular contraction is very effective in eliminating the false negatives. This can often be helpful with an edematous or lymphatically compromised lower extremity due to extrinsic pressure the edema produces on the vein.[40]

4. Parana maneuver. A variation to the active muscular contraction, a standing patient is asked to slightly rock forward or backward, to offset standing equilibrium, to engage the calf muscles (isometric contraction). This can also be achieved by asking the patient to shift their weight slightly from one leg to the other. This maneuver is more closely related to the muscular changes that occur with walking and is gaining preference for producing and testing flux and reflux in phlebologic patients.

Although challenging, with practice, this technique can also be very useful.

5. Automatic cuff devices. The use of blood pressure-type cuffs to facilitate a compression augmentation is another method to determine reflux. This is the commonly used method for research and investigative studies. Some sonographers suggest this to be cumbersome for routine use in daily practice, while others prefer them from an ergonomic standpoint and, with foot pedals, they are quite easy to use. Although inflation and deflation are common terms for the equipment, for reflux testing, a rapid, large caliber deflation port, which assists in mimicking the diastole following compression, is key. Several authors have indicated use of pressures from 80 to 120 mmHg depending on the segment of the leg being tested.[37, 46] Another key consideration as described by Partsch and Partsch[56] includes the relationship between pressure and valve closure which obviously impacts on reflux times.

6. Repeated or successive augmentation at the same location. This concept relates to the capacitance of the varicose bed. By using repeated augmentation in quick succession, capacitance of the distal venous bed is reduced similar to the effect of lowered venous pressure that occurs with walking. As one would expect, this results in a decreased amount of reflux in each successive augmentation. Therefore, in order to obtain an accurate duplex reflux tracing, a small time delay should be used for documentation and interpretation purposes, if repeated augmentations occur.

7. Proximal augmentation. Although in many ways, proximal augmentation is similar to a Valsalva maneuver, applying proximal pressure to 'force' blood down the vein the wrong way to test the valve is less than accurate. Many, question its validity and accuracy especially for superficial determinations. Van Bemmelen *et al.* stated, 'This study emphasizes that the maneuvers to elicit closure of the valve are at least as important as the methods to monitor reflux flow itself. ... Manual compression of the supine limb proximal to the transducer site *did not result in closure of the valve but rather in reflux during the entire compression* followed by cessation of flow ... the correct and consistent

translation of reflux into valve incompetence is a prerequisite for the understanding of pathophysiologic characteristics of veins.'[46] Further, van Bemmelen states, 'reverse velocities greater than 30 cm/sec result in value closure' adding that 'the use of proximal compression … cannot lead to reliable, objective results'.[57] *Therefore, the authors believe that proximal compression should be avoided as a testing method for reflux.*

The above techniques are useful and complementary, while also having some limitations. A full understanding of the advantages and limitations of each allows the skillful examiner to use them in a complementary method in various situations to facilitate understanding reflux, and the true clinical picture.

Other general considerations and terms for venous duplex scanning

When pathology is present, compressibility, appearance of thrombus, location, and extent should be documented. Focal calf pain will generally require evaluation of the localized region. To better visualize a thrombus, accessing its extent in both longitudinal and short axis is helpful, while using both B-mode and color flow for complementary information. Comparison with prior relevant imaging studies may also prove helpful.

Documentation

As with other medical procedures, permanent documentation of each diagnostic study is required. Specifics vary based on local or state laws in the United States (and across the world). Generally, however, a duplex examination should be thought of as an x-ray and therefore archived and stored for seven years. The general trend is moving away from hard copy, and being replaced with digital storage. Proper storage, identification, and cross-referencing techniques are required for any media, video clips, digital or hard copy prints, etc., regardless of format.

A written (or electronic) request is required to initiate the study, and should provide for the medical necessity of the examination, including the indications noted earlier in this chapter. This needs to be initiated by a physician or other appropriate provider (i.e. nurse practitioner or physician's assistant). Other information on elements to include in a report, including timelines, are part of the reporting process discussed more fully in Chapter 6.

All technical findings should be recorded on a worksheet and provided along with the recorded images to the physician for use in preparing a final report. This includes the concept of a vein map (discussed elsewhere) and should be part of the permanent record of the examination. The interpreting and referring physician should be alerted when immediate medical attention is indicated based on the examination findings.

An overview Adapted from ICAVL for the Documentation for Deep Vein Thrombosis and Chronic Venous Insufficiency

Below is a summary of the minimum hard copy documentation requirements for venous testing for ICAVL accreditation. Please note that these are two separate and distinct tests and only one test should need to be performed on the patient based on their symptoms. Also additional images may be needed for insurance reimbursement if the patient is seeking possible treatment.

Testing for Thrombosis and Patency (DVT)

- Representative gray scale images with and without transverse transducer compressions
  - ▶ Common Femoral Vein
  - ▶ Saphenofemoral Junction
  - ▶ Proximal Femoral Vein
  - ▶ Mid Femoral Vein
  - ▶ Distal Femoral Vein
  - ▶ Popliteal Vein
  - ▶ Posterior Tibial Veins
  - ▶ Peroneal Veins
  - ▶ Additional images to document areas of suspected thrombosis
  - ▶ Additional images if required by the laboratory protocol
- Representative spectral Doppler waveforms in longitudinal axis (showing variations with respirations and/or manual flow augmentation)
  - ▶ Right and left Common Femoral Veins
  - ▶ Popliteal Vein
  - ▶ Additional waveforms if required by the laboratory protocol

Testing for Lower Extermity Reflux (Venous Insufficiency)

- Representative gray scale images with and without transverse transducer compressions
  - ▶ Common Femoral Vein
  - ▶ Saphenofemoral Junction
  - ▶ Mid Femoral Vein
  - ▶ Great Saphenous Vein (GSV)
  - ▶ Popliteal Vein
  - ▶ Small Saphenous Vein (SSV)
  - ▶ Additional images to document areas of suspected thrombus
  - ▶ Additional images if required by the laboratory protocol

Respresentative spectral doppler waveforms in longitudinal axis (showing baseline and during reflux producing maneuvers)

  - ▶ Common Femoral Vein
  - ▶ Saphenofemoral Junction
  - ▶ Great Saphenous Vein
  - ▶ Femoral Vein
  - ▶ Popliteal Vein
  - ▶ Small Saphenous Vein
  - ▶ Suspected areas of reflux including spectral Doppler waveforms
  - ▶ Additional images if required by the laboratory protocol

   In addition to the above images, you may want to include documentation of the following for insurance reimbursement:
   - *Vein diameters in the GSV and SSV*
   - *Reflux duration times (Sec or msec)*

References:

2010 ICAVL Standards, Part V (www.icavl.org)

2010 SVU Lower Extremity Venous Insufficiency Evaluation (www.svunet.org)

Figure 5.35

Overview on the Process for Performing a Lower Extremity Venous Reflux Examination

Purpose

- To evaluate the deep and superficial veins for evidence of valvular incompetence.
- This examination is not urgent or emergent since the physician has already examined the patient and determined that they do not have the signs/symptoms for DVT.

Steps

- Introduce myself and explain the test to be performed. Answer any questions.
- Have the patient change into a gown or shorts.
- Examine the legs for obvious signs of venous disease – varicose veins, skin changes, edema, stasis, ulcers, etc. This can give you a clue as to what you may find during the exam.
- Ask the patient about family or personal history of DVT or PE, previous vein surgery, and current symptoms (painful, achy, heavy, tired legs, throbbing, restless legs, calf cramps, etc). If female ask about any miscarriages.
- Have the patient lie down supine with the table in a slight reverse Trendelenburg.
    - Assess the deep veins (CFV, SFJ, FV and PopV) using probe compressions along the entire vein to make sure the walls coapt completely.
    - Assess the spectral Doppler waveforms in the CFV bilaterally, noting whether the waveforms are similar which is normal, or different which could be from a proximal obstruction.
    - If a proximal obstruction is suspected, try to assess the iliac veins and IVC.
    - Document images showing compressibility at CFV, SFJ, mid-FV and PopV, as well as the CFV waveforms.
    - *If an acute DVT is found*, interrupt the reflux study continue with a complete DVT protocol to assess the deep veins in more detail, including the deep calf veins.
- Have the patient stand up.
    - Remember that the patient's weight should be on the opposite leg of the one that is being examined.
    - Assess the deep veins for reflux (CFV, SFJ, FV and PopV) using distal augmentation. The Valsalva maneuver can be used at the CFV and SFJ.
    - Document images showing spectral Doppler at CFV, SFJ, mid-FV and PopV.
- With the patient's back to you:
    - Assess the SSV for diameter, reflux and compressibility from the popliteal crease to the ankle, looking and assessing for any large tributaries or perforators that come into or come out of the SSV.
    - Document images showing compressibility, diameter and spectral Doppler at proximal SSV (popliteal crease) and mid SSV.
    - Look for the thigh extension and vein of Giacomini. If found, assess for the diameter and reflux.
    - Document images of diameter and spectral Doppler.
- Have the patient turn around and face you.
    - Assess the GSV for diameter, reflux and compressibility from the SFJ to the proximal calf, looking for any areas in the GSV where the vein becomes larger or smaller due to tributaries or perforators.
    - Document images showing compressibility, diameter and spectral Doppler at the proximal, mid- and distal GSV in the thigh and the proximal GSV in the calf.
    - Assess the anterior accessory saphenous vein (AASV) at or near the SFJ for the diameter and reflux.
    - Document images of diameter and spectral Doppler.
    - Assess any other large tributaries and perforators in the thigh for diameter and reflux.
    - Document the diameter and spectral Doppler for any abnormal findings.

Figure 5.36 *(Continued)*

Overview on the Process for Performing a Lower Extremity Venous Reflux Examination

- Have the patient sit down and dangle lower legs.
  - Assess the perforating veins in the calf for diameter and reflux.
  - Document the diameter and spectral Doppler for any abnormal findings.
- After performing all of the above, ask yourself:
  - Did I determine where the varicosities are coming from?
  - For example, if a patient presents with varicosities on the lateral calf and the GSV, SSV, AASV, etc., are all normal, have you done the exam? The answer is No! Go to the varicosities and scan proximally to try to determine the origin of reflux. *This is similar to a DVT exam, where after looking at all of the necessary veins you examine the area of pain.*

Tips and Tricks

- If you are having difficultly identifying the GSV at the SFJ, start at the mid thigh and locate the GSV within the saphenous fascia, then move proximally to the inguinal fold.
- If you are having difficulty identifying the SSV, start at the mid-posterior calf and locate the SSV within the fascia, then move proximally to the popliteal fossa.
- The AASV can be identified by its relationship with the deep vessels. It is usually found directly above the femoral vein and artery (alignment sign), whereas the GSV is medial to these deep vessels.
- Do not concern yourself with every tributary, concentrate on tributaries that are the same size or larger than the truncal vein it is connecting with.
- If a vein measures less than 2 mm in diameter, it is not necessary to perform a spectral Doppler.
- Remember that perforating veins go down to the deep veins whereas tributaries/branches go up to varicosities (epifascial).
- Do not spend a great deal of time on perforating veins less than 3 mm in diameter.
- Use color Doppler to help locate the best area for placing the sample gate.
- If an obstruction in the abdominal veins (iliacs or IVC) is suspected, measure the CFV with and without Valsalva. The CFV should increase in size with Valsalva.
- If reflux is found, measure the duration in seconds or milliseconds.
- Be sure to document normal, as well as abnormal findings, in the main truncal veins.
- Diameter measurements are usually taken in a transverse view, anterior to posterior walls.
- Spectral Doppler waveforms are usually taken in a longitudinal view.
- If a patient is unable to stand, have them lean against the table and place their buttocks on the edge of the table. If they have a walker with a seat, they can sit on the edge of the seat with their feet on the floor. Be sure to note on the worksheet if the patient's position varies from the standard protocol.
- If the patient is having trouble performing the Valsalva maneuver, ask them to put the tip of their thumb in their mouth, create a seal, and blow like they are blowing up a balloon.

Figure 5.36

REFERENCES

1. Bergan J. *The Vein Book.* Burlington, MA: Elsevier Academic Press, 2007.
2. Gerotziafas GT, Samama MM. Prophylaxis of venous thromboembolism in medical patients. *Current Opinion in Pulmonary Medicine* 2004; 10: 356–65.
3. Anderson FA, Audet AM. *Preventing deep vein thrombosis and pulmonary embolism. A practical guide to evaluation and improvement.* Worcester, MA: Center for Outcomes Research, University of Massachusetts Medical Center, 1998.
4. O'Meara PM, Kaufmann EE. Prophylaxis for venous thromboembolism in total hip arthroplasty: a review. *Orthopedics* 1990; **13**: 173–8.
5. Sandler DA, Martin JF. Autopsy proven pulmonary embolism in hospital patients: are we detecting enough deep vein thrombosis? *Journal of Royal Society of Medicine* 1989; **82**: 203–5.

6. Kalodiki E, Stvrtinova V, Allegra C *et al.* Prevention of venous thromboembolism – International Consensus Statement. *International Angiology* 1997; **16**: 3–38.

7. Sandford DA, Kelly D, Rhee SJ *et al.* Importance of phasicity in detection of proximal iliac vein thrombosis with venous duplex examination. *Journal of Vascular Ultrasound* 2011; **35**: 150–2.

8. De Maeseneer M, Pichot O, Cavezzi A *et al.* Duplex ultrasound investigation of the veins of the lower limbs after treatment for varicose veins. UIP Consensus Document. *European Journal of Vascular and Endovascular Surgery* 2011; **42**: 89–102.

9. ACP Duplex ultrasound imaging of lower extremities veins in chronic venous disease, exclusive of deep venous thrombosis: guidelines for performance and interpretation of studies. Accessed August 2010. Available from: www.phlebology.org.

10. Society of Vascular Ultrasound. Vascular technology professional performance guidelines: lower extremity venous insufficiency evaluation. Accessed November 2010. Available from: www.svunet.org.

11. ACR AIUM SRU. Practice guideline for the performance of peripheral venous ultrasound examination. Accessed September 2010. Available from www.acr.org.

12. ICAVL. Standards for accreditation in non-invasive vascular testing, Part II, Peripheral venous testing. Accessed November 2009. Available from: www.icavl.org.

13. ACR. Practice guidelines for performing and interpreting diagnostic ultrasound examinations, rev 2011. Accessed January 2012. Available from: www.acr.org.

14. Mauriello J. Popliteal vein compression. Abstract from 25th Annual Congress of the American College of Phlebology, Los Angeles, November, 2011.

15. Lane RJ, Cuzzilla ML, Haris RA, Phillips MN. Popliteal vein compression syndrome: obesity, venous disease and the popliteal connection. *Phlebology* 2009; **24**: 201–20.

16 Walsh JC, Bergan JJ, Beeman S, Comer TP. Femoral venous reflux abolished by greater saphenous vein stripping. *Annals of Vascular Surgery* 1994; **8**: 566–570.

17 Sales CM, Bilof ML, Petrillo KS, Luka NL. Correction of lower extremity deep venous incompetence by ablation of superficial venous reflux. *Annals of Vascular Surgery* 1996; **10**: 186–189.

18. Labropoulos N, Delis K, Nicolaides AN *et al.* The role of the distribution and anatomic extent of reflux in the development of signs and symptoms in chronic venous insufficiency. *Journal of Vascular Surgery* 1996; **23**: 504–10.

19. Zamboni P, Cisno C, Marchetti F *et al.* Reflux elimination without any ablation or disconnection of the saphenous vein. A haemodynamic model for venous surgery. *European Journal of Vascular and Endovascular Surgery* 2001; **21**: 361–9.

20. Kostas T, Ioannou C, Touloupakis E *et al.* Recurrent varicose veins after surgery: a new appraisal of a common and complex problem in vascular surgery. *European Journal of Vascular and Endovascular Surgery* 2004; **27**: 275–82.

21. Creton D, Pare EC. Diameter reduction of the proximal long saphenous vein after ablation of a distal incompetent tributary. *Dermatologic Surgery* 1999; **25**: 394–8.

22. Somjen GM, Royle JP, Fell G *et al.* Venous reflux patterns in the popliteal fossa. *Journal of Cardiovascular Surgery* 1992; **33**: 85–91.

23. Zygmunt J. What's new in duplex scanning of the venous system. *Perspectives in Vascular Surgery and Endovascular Therapy* 2009; **21**: 94–104.

24. Lurie F, Kistner R, Perrin M *et al.* Invasive treatment of deep venous disease. A UIP Consensus. *International Angiology* 2010; **29**: 199–204.

25. Francheschi C. *Theorie et pratique de la cure conservatrice et hemodynamique de l'insuffisance veineuse en ambulatiore.* Precy-sous-Thil: Editions de l' Armancon, 1988.

26. Obermeyer A, Garzon K. Sourcing of superficial reflux in venous leg ulcers by duplex ultrasound. *Journal of Vascular Surgery* 2010; **52**: 1255–61.

27. Blomgren L, Johansson G, Dahlberg-Åkerman A *et al.* Changes in superficial and perforating vein reflux after varicose vein surgery. *Journal of Vascular Surgery* 2005; **42**: 315–20.

28. Gloviczki P, Comerota AJ, Dalsing MC *et al.* The care of patients with varicose veins and

associated chronic venous diseases: clinical practice guidelines of the Society for Vascular Surgery and the American Venous Forum. *Journal of Vascular Surgery* 2011; **53**: 2S–48S.

29. Malgor RD, Labropolous N. Diagnosis of follow-up of varicose veins with duplex ultrasound: how and why? Phlebology 2012; **27** (Suppl 1): 10–15.

30. Foldes M, Blackburn M, Hogan J *et al.* Standing versus supine positioning in venous reflux evaluation. *Journal of Vascular Technology* 1991; **15**: 321–4.

31. Houle M, Neuhardt D, Straight N *et al.* Differences in saphenous vein reflux detection according to patient positioning. Abstract UIP, Monaco, 2009.

32. Labropolous N, Kokkosis AA, Spentzouris G *et al.* The distribution and significance of varicosities in the saphenous trunks. *Journal of Vascular Surgery* 2010; **51**: 96–103.

33. Chiesa R, Marone EM, Limoni C *et al.* Chronic venous disorders: correlation between visible signs, symptoms, and presence of functional disease. *Journal of Vascular Surgery* 2007; **46**: 322–30.

34. Pieri A, Gatti M, Santini M *et al.* Ultrasonographic anatomy of the deep veins of the lower extremity. *Journal of Vascular Technology* 2002; **26**: 201–11.

35. Labropoulos N, Delis K, Nicolaides AN *et al.* The role of the distribution and anatomic extent of reflux in the development of signs and symptoms in chronic venous insufficiency. *Journal of Vascular Surgery* 1996; **23**: 504–10.

36. Carandina S, Mari C, DePalma M *et al.* Varicose vein stripping vs haemodynamic correction (CHIVA): a long term randomized trial. *European Journal of Vascular and Endovascular Surgery* 2008; **35**: 230–7.

37. Labropoulos N, Leon L, Kwon S *et al.* Study of the venous reflux progression. *Journal of Vascular Surgery* 2005; **41**: 291–5.

38. Pittaluga, P, *et al.* Classification of saphenous refluxes : implications for treatment, *Phlebology* 2008; 23: 2-9

39. Bernardini *et al.* Development of primary superficial venous insufficiency: the ascending theory. *Annals of Vascular Surgery* 2010; 24: 709-720

40. Labropoulos N, Tiongson J, Pryor L *et al.* Definition of venous reflux in lower-extremity veins. *Journal of Vascular Surgery* 2003; **38**: 793–8.

41. Coleridge-Smith P, Labropoulos N, Partsch H *et al.* Duplex ultrasound investigation of the veins in chronic venous disease of the lower limbs. UIP Consensus Document. Part I Basic principles. *European Journal of Vascular and Endovascular Surgery* 2006; **31**: 83–92.

42. Jutley R, Cadle I, Cross K. Preoperative assessment of primary varicose veins: a duplex study of venous incompetence. *European Journal of Vascular and Endovascular Surgery* 2001; **21**: 370–3.

43. Tarrant G, Clarke J. Differences in venous function of the lower limb by time of day: a comparison of chronic venous insufficiency between an afternoon and a morning appointment by duplex ultrasound. *Journal for Vascular Ultrasound* 2008; **32**: 187–92.

44. Maurins U, Hoffmann B, Lösch C *et al.* Distribution and prevalence of reflux in the superficial and deep venous system in the general population – results from the Bonn Vein Study, Germany. *Journal of Vascular Surgery* 2008; **48**: 680–7.

45. Stuart W, Lee A, Allan P *et al.* Most incompetent calf perforating veins are found in association with superficial venous reflux. *Journal of Vascular Surgery* 2001; **43**: 774–8.

46. van Bemmelen P, Bedford G, Beach K, Strandness DE. Quantitative segmental evaluation of venous valvular reflux with duplex ultrasound scanning. *Journal of Vascular Surgery* 1989; **10**: 425–31.

47. Labropolous, N, Zygmunt, J. Letter to the Editor - Clinical Significance of Standing versus Reversed Trendlenburg Position for the Diagnosis of Lower-Extremity Venous Reflux in the Great Saphenous Vein. *Journal for Vascular Ultrasound* 2012; 36(2): 159–160.

48. Pemble L. Lower extremity venous cross-sectional area changes associated with pregnancy. *Journal for Vascular Ultrasound* 2006; **30**: 75–80.

49. Meissner M, Moneta G, Burnand K *et al.* The hemodynamics and diagnosis of venous disease *Journal of Vascular Surgery* 2007; **46**: 4S–24S.

50. Tarrant G, Clarke J. Differences in venous function of the lower limb by time of day: a comparison of chronic venous insufficiency between an afternoon and a morning appointment by duplex ultrasound. *Journal for Vascular Ultrasound* 2008; **32**: 187–92.

51. Lurie F, Comerota A, Eklof B *et al.* Multicenter assessment of venous reflux by duplex ultrasound. *Journal of Vascular Surgery* 2012; **55**: 437–45.

52 Gibson K, Meissner M, Wright D. Great saphenous vein diameter does not correlate with worsening quality of life scores in patients with great saphenous vein incompetence. *Journal of Vascular Surgery* 2012 [Epub ahead of print].

53. Lurie F, Kistner R, Eklof B, Kessler D. Mechanism of venous valve closure and role of the valve in circulation: a new concept. *Journal of Vascular Surgery* 2003; **38**: 955–61.

54. Labropoulos N, Tassiopoulos A, Bhatti A, Leon L. Development of reflux in the perforator veins in limbs with primary venous disease. *Journal of Vascular Surgery* 2006; **43**: 558–62.

55. Beckwith T, Richardson G, Sheldon M, Clarke G. A correlation between blood flow volume and ultrasonic Doppler wave forms in the study of valve efficiency. *Phlebology* 1993; **8**: 12–16.

56. Partsch B, Partsch H. Calf compression pressure required to achieve venous closure from supine to standing positions. *Journal of Vascular Surgery* 2005; **42**: 734–8.

57. van Bemmelen P, Beach K, Bedford G, Strandness DE. The mechanism of venous value closure. *Archives of Surgery* 1990; **125**: 617–619.

6

Ultrasound performance, interpretation, documentation and reporting, credentialing, and accreditation

Introduction

The following section is based primarily on the practices, guidelines, and standard of care in the United States. This is not meant to suggest that standards, procedures, and guidelines are absent in other countries. These concepts are certainly foundational and transferable to anyone practicing the phlebologic arts. In the authors' discussions and observations with international colleagues, many of these same concepts are followed diligently throughout the world.

In the United States, ultrasound examinations are performed primarily by sonographers and this represents the technical component of the examination. Following acquisition of the images, the findings (images and worksheets) are interpreted by qualified physicians, rendering a diagnosis with a report generated, which represents the professional component. These two parts make up a global or complete ultrasound examination. In other parts of the world (as well as in the United States), ultrasounds can and are performed and interpreted by a physician. Regardless of who actually performs or interprets the ultrasound, methodologies and standardization of processes are required. Primarily, these standardizations are for quality and accuracy assurance. Additional reasons for these processes include reimbursement and legal issues for which adequate documentation of the medical procedure represent the standard of care. As noted in some of the references in the development of this chapter, the guidelines and protocols are suggested as good practice recommendations.

They are not inflexible rules or requirements of practice and are not intended, nor should they be used, to establish a legal standard of care … The ultimate judgment regarding the propriety of any specific procedure or course of action must be made by the physician … However, a practitioner who employs an approach substantially different from these guidelines is advised to document in the patient record information sufficient to explain the approach taken.[1]

In the United States, two- and four-year college level ultrasound schools have developed to promote proper education and training for the performance of diagnostic ultrasound by sonographers. Interestingly, several of the ultrasound credentialing organizations are discussing moving away from 'on-the-job'-type training which was the foundation of the ultrasound community in the 1980s and 1990s. As with other advancements, this is a step towards formalization which should be readily embraced. Other steps at standardization include the development and implementation of standardized protocols, registry level testing, professional development with continuing educational requirements, and accreditation organizations. Historically, these steps were voluntary and done in order to pro-mote excellence and quality as part of the honorable responsibility of health-care providers. Recently, the INVEST study, carried out under the umbrella of the American Venous Forum brought to light incon-sistencies in protocol and training, and therefore issues regarding repeatability and reproducibility of venous reflux examinations are becoming more understood.[2]

In more recent times, diagnostic ultrasound has become recognized as a revenue-producing service. Furthermore, medical interventions are based on the results of these ultrasound investigations, not only with regard to quality, but additionally with regard to payment for services and the resulting interventions. Efforts to maintain the quality of care with respect to ultrasound are becoming com-monplace. Patients and physicians alike look to understand the quality of care being delivered since medical decisions and treatment are based on these sonographic examinations.

Although not discussed openly, there exists a dichotomy between accuracy and the financial impact of the results in a procedure-driven reim-bursement model and potential for abuse exists. The potential for over-estimation of disease by those driven by financial gain is recognized, and hopefully minimal. Although this may be per-ceived to reside on the shoulders of the interpret-ing physician, other areas of concern exist. The mobile ultrasound service or the sonographer who is 'employed' by the physician or hospital who believes or may be pressured to 'find disease' for a physician or clinic so procedures can be performed, and income generated, also potentially have a con-flict of interest. Although these circumstances are outliers, the potential exists all the same and stand-ardization, documentation, and protocols will help to minimize these issues. Additionally, Medicare and many of the private insurance carriers in the United States have adopted policies which limit payment only to those people or facilities which meet and maintain minimum standards. These standards and policies have experienced a natural evolution, are not static, and it is an incumbent responsibility of the conscientious practitioner to stay abreast of these evolving processes. In this section, a review of some current concepts regard-ing the performance of quality ultrasound will be reviewed.

There are several professional organizations in the United States which provide performance guidelines, recommendations for protocols, posi-tion statements or that offer credentialing for an individual or facility. These organizations include but are not limited to the following.

Professional societies

American College of Radiology (ACR) www.acr.org

American College of Phlebology (ACP) www.phlebology.org

American Institute of Ultrasound in Medicine (AIUM) www.aium.org

Society of Vascular Ultrasound (SVU) www.suvnet.org

Society of Diagnostic Medical Sonography (SMDS) www.sdms.org

Credentialing organizations

American Registry for Diagnostic Medical Sonographers (ARDMS) www.ardms.org

Cardiovascular Credentialing International (CCI) www.cci-online.org

Intersocietal Comission for Accreditation (IAC) vascular division (formerly ICAVL) www.intersocietal.org/vascular

Performance

Diagnostic ultrasound studies should be performed by those medical professionals with the training, knowledge, and experience of ultrasound and its limitations. Physician responsibilities in this regard pertain to those who supervise, perform, and/or interpret diagnostic sonography. It should be noted that qualifications to perform ultrasound studies and the qualifications to interpret ultrasound stud-ies are similar, but not identical. In this scenario, the physician should be licenced, with a thorough understanding of venous anatomy, physiology, hemodynamics, and clinical manifestations of ve-nous disease, knowledge of ultrasound physics, indi-cations for testing, criteria for diagnosis of pathology, documentation requirements, technical limitations, and an understanding of the skills necessary to perform these studies. Qualification is typically demonstrated through fellowship or training programs which include involvement in the supervision and/or performance of a minimum number of ultrasound procedures. This ranges from 300 to 500 or more with different organizations and includes specific recommendations for maintenance of competence and continuing medical education requirements.

For sonographers, the qualification for performance includes criteria of documentation of training and experience and is typically demonstrated by achievement of certification with one of the internationally recognized certifying bodies in a particular field of interest. Notwithstanding that credentialing is a valid and worthy accomplishment, it does not guarantee that studies will be performed at the levels we are speaking about here. Ultrasound examinations are completely technique- and operator-dependent, and a recent study noted that 'measuring the technical competence is challenging'.[3] These certifications also require continuing medical education to remain in good standing. Currently, there are legislative movements to require state licensure of sonographers. There are mixed thoughts regarding this in both the sonography and legislative communities, as to whether this will provide stronger incentive for competence. Below is a brief listing of licencing activities by state, this is a worthy but evolving issue.

- Oregon: licencing began July 1, 2010, with a provisional licence available until 2014
- New Mexico: law passed in 2009, but implementation has been delayed
- West Virginia: a bill has been drafted and expected to hit state legislators in 2011
- New Jersey: a bill was submitted to the New Jersey Senate, but did not receive support from the sonography community and these efforts appear to have been halted.[4]

All interpreting physicians (medical staff) and practicing technologist (technical staff) must be adequately trained and experienced to interpret and perform non-invasive vascular testing, respectively.[5]

Credentialing of sonographers for vascular studies is typically recognized with the acquisition of the following designations: registered vascular technologist (RVT), registered vascular specialist (RVS), or, for venous exams, the newly developed registered phlebology sonographer (RPhS), credentials that can be earned from ARDMS and CCI for the latter two credentials. Physician training is commonly demonstrated by specialty and fellowship training, the acquisition of the credentials above or additionally the Registered Physician in Vascular Interpretation (RPVI) offered by ARDMS. More information on each of these will be described later in this chapter.

Key guidelines

Orders

Diagnostic ultrasound studies are performed upon written or electronic request for the study. The request must come from a physician or other properly licenced health-care provider, e.g. physician's assistant or nurse practitioner. The request should demonstrate the medical necessity of the examination. With regard to venous evaluations both venous obstruction (deep vein thrombosis, DVT) and venous insufficiency (reflux) have individual protocols, and each require a valid indication.

Indications

Documentation that satisfies medical necessity includes: (1) signs and symptoms and/or (2) relevant history, including known diagnoses. Additional information regarding the specific reason for the examination or a provisional diagnosis.[1] By way of example, a common list of indications for peripheral venous examinations include, but are not limited to:

1) Evaluation of venous thromboembolic disease or venous obstruction
2) Preoperative evaluation of venous insufficiency
3) Visible varicose veins
4) Venous ulcer
5) Pain, edema, or discoloration including skin changes
6) End of anticoagulation regime for determination of residual venous thrombosis.

The Society of Vascular Ultrasound's professional performance guidelines are highly recommended and several key elements of that document are paraphrased below.[6]

Guideline 2. Patient assessment and physical examination: a patient assessment must be performed before the ultrasound examination. This assessment includes a limited or focused physical examination to include observation and localization of the signs and symptoms of venous disease.

Guideline 3. The information gathered during the examination is analyzed during the course of the evaluation to ensure that sufficient data are provided to the physician to direct the patient's management and render a final diagnosis.

Guideline 5. Present the documentation of diagnostic images, data, explanations, and technical worksheet to the interpreting physician for interpretation and rendering of a diagnosis.

Documentation and interpretation

Documentation should follow the written protocols of the facility performing the examination. For studies performed in a physician's office, this still applies, and a written protocol should be strictly adhered to for quality control measures. Documentation should provide sufficient images and other information to allow for proper interpretation of the examination. This could include: (1) gray-scale images; (2) Doppler wave forms; (3) velocity or time measurements; and (4) other measurements or images as required by the protocol. Although hard-copy documentation was historically required, digital storage of images and records has become the preferred method. As with other medical documentation, seven years of properly archived storage is recommended for various reasons.

Documentation typically includes the technical worksheets and notes made during the examination, but also the interpretation of the test results. Interpretation may or may not include a technical impression prior to the final physician interpretation. However, if a technical impression is part of the process, this should be part of written protocols. The physician review of images and technical worksheets should be performed within 2 days and a final verified signed report should be prepared within 4 days. These details should also be part of a written

protocol.[2] Protocols should delineate methods for communication for urgent or life-threatening findings. Also, reasons for a suboptimal, incomplete, or otherwise limited examination should be included in any instance when variance from the standard protocol occurs. In any instance when the protocol is not followed, this information needs to be well documented and reported. The report is the final interpretation and is part of the patient's medical records, which is a legal document and should be retrievable and/or reproducible for review.

Scanning and documentation protocols

Regardless of the place of service, diagnostic ultrasound examinations should be done following the written protocol of the hospital, diagnostic laboratory, mobile service, or physician's office in which the study is performed. Protocols are the written documents that detail the procedural steps followed when performing a certain study or examination.

In theory, this ensures that no matter who is performing the study, sufficient data (e.g. images and/or other information) are collected on every patient each time the study is performed. If it is not possible to follow the written protocol, documentation should provide explanation of the reason or reasons for the limited or incomplete examination. These protocols should be printed out in hard-copy form and placed in a conspicuous place within the facility, office, or vascular laboratory.

Every type of ultrasound examination that is performed should have a written protocol and this should be adhered to in every case. In the phlebology setting, two types of ultrasound examinations are most commonly performed: (1) a study for deep vein thrombosis or obstruction or (2) a venous insufficiency examination that includes both the deep and superficial systems. More recently, additional investigation into the external iliacs, common iliacs, and distal inferior vena cava (IVC) are being performed more frequently. It is mandatory that the venous insufficiency examination includes at a minimum evaluation of the deep veins of the thigh. One key element in the venous insufficiency examination is to find the source of reflux in the patient's varicosities, and the examination should not be considered complete until this is well documented.

Basic elements

There are certain basic elements included in a written protocol and described in the interpretation, which include:

- Name of examination
- Purpose: general reason the study is being performed (to evaluate …)
- Indications: clinical signs and symptoms or relevant history (including known diagnoses) that validate the reason for performing the study
- Contraindications and limitations
- Equipment utilized: name of ultrasound machine and type of probe
- Examination technique: description of which veins will be studied and which techniques will be used
- Elements of proper technique
- The anatomic extent of the examination, i.e. a complete examination includes evaluation of the entire course of each vein listed in the protocol
- Variations on differences between a bilateral or unilateral studies, i.e. for a unilateral study, the contralateral common femoral vein should be evaluated
- Patient preparation and positioning
- Variations in the protocol for repeated or recurring limited examinations (a limited examination is typically a subset of steps that are present in a complete examination). A separate protocol should be considered for repetitive limited examinations with indications, etc.
- Documentation acquisition: the protocol contains a list of images to be documented, even if the test is normal, serial image documentation is required. Also, a description that provides for the additional images or waveforms that demonstrate the severity, location, and extent of the pathology found on the examination is required for abnormal findings.

Sample protocols and technical worksheets

As noted earlier, separate protocols for DVT and reflux document the differences in these examinations,[7] and a sample of each is provided for the reader. These should be examined closely, altered or adjusted during implementation, to be fully understood. Additionally, examples of technical worksheets accompany each examination (Figures 6.1, 6.2, 6.3, and 6.4, and see Box 8.2 in Chapter 8).

Credentialing and accreditation

Credentialing

The role of the vascular technologist is to perform a wide range of non-invasive vascular studies which assist physicians in the diagnosis and treatment of a wide variety of disorders affecting the vascular system (excluding the heart) (www.suvnet.org).

Credentialing in vascular ultrasound is available from two main organizations: (1) the American Registry for Diagnostic Medical Sonography and (2) the Cardiovascular Credentialing International, additionally vascular credentialing (VS) can be acheived through the American College of Radiology (ACR).

Most employers prefer to hire credentialed vascular technologists. Many insurance carriers are now requiring that vascular studies be performed by credentialed vascular technologists or in accredited vascular laboratories in order to receive reimbursement.

Registered Vascular Technologist

The American Registry for Diagnostic Medical Sonography, incorporated in June 1975, is an independent, non-profit organization that administers examinations and awards credentials in the areas of diagnostic medical sonography, diagnostic cardiac sonography, vascular interpretation, and vascular technology. There are currently approximately 19 500 registered vascular technologists (RVT). Contact information: www.ardms.org; 51 Monroe Street, Plaza East One, Rockville, MD 20850-2400, USA; Telephone: 001 301 738 8401 or 001 800 541 9754.

To earn the RVT credential, applicants are required to pass two comprehensive examinations: (1) Sonography Principles and Instrumentation (SPI) examination and (2) Vascular Technology specialty examination.

The SPI examination is 2 hours long and contains approximately 120 multiple-choice questions. It will test basic physical principles and instrumentation

LE Venous Duplex for DVT

Examination

Lower Extremity Venous Duplex for DVT

Purpose

To assess venous anatomy and venous flow patterns utilizing real time B-mode ultrasound imaging and Doppler spectrum flow analysis to determine the patency, hemodynamics of flow, and anatomic abnormalities of the veins.

Equipment Utilized

- Duplex Ultrasound machine with Spectral Doppler, Color Doppler and B-mode capabilities
- 5-12 MHz linear probe

Patient Preparation and Positioning

- Introduction to patient and a brief explanation of the examination
- Obtain pertinent patient history
- Brief examination of the lower extremities for signs of DVT- edema, tenderness, inflammation, erythema
- Patient puts on shorts or drape to allow for examination of entire leg
- Patient is placed in a supine position with the limbs externally rotated 10-15 degree reversed Trendelenburg position

Examination Technique

- Study may be unilateral or bilateral. If unilateral, a contralateral common femoral vein (CFV) spectral waveform must be documented
- Equipment gain and display settings should be optimized to provide the best possible B-mode images; color flow Doppler is utilized to assist in identifying vessels
- Spectral waveforms are obtained using a Doppler angle of sixty degrees or less, keeping the cursor aligned parallel to the vessel wall
- Transverse probe compression maneuvers are performed every 2 cm along entire vein to test for DVT
- The entire lower extremity venous system should be assessed using both imaging and Doppler interrogation, obtaining hardcopy documentation as required by the Documentation Acquisition portion of this protocol

Documentation Acquisition

The following documentation must be obtained with additional documentation of questionable and abnormal or incidental findings.

- B-mode images with <u>probe compression maneuvers every 2 cm</u> using split screen (transverse):
  - CFV
  - SFJ
  - Proximal FV
  - Mid FV
  - Distal FV
  - Pop V
  - Posterior Tibial Veins
  - Peroneal Veins
  - Inferior Vena Cava (IVC), External Iliac Vein (EIV) and calf muscle veins are documented when necessary
  - Additional representative images of areas of suspected thrombosis
- Spectral Doppler waveforms with <u>distal compression of the limb</u> (longitudinal):
  - CFV
  - Pop V
- Record all findings on the technologist's worksheet.

Special Considerations

- For obese patients, it may be necessary to use a lower frequency transducer
- For patients that have open draining ulcers, it may be necessary to use a probe cover
- Patients with severe edema that can impede accurate assessment of the calf vessels

Reviewed

Date: _____ Medical Director: _____ Technical Director: _____

Figure 6.1 Protocol for deep vein evaluation.

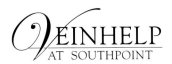

Lower Extremity Venous Duplex

Patient Name:_____ Date: _____

Referring M.D. _____ Study Performed by: _____

Indications: _____ Prior Exam: Date/Results _____

History:
- ⭕ Swelling
- ⭕ Smoking
- ⭕ Chemo/XRT

- ⭕ CHF
- ⭕ Prior DVT
- ⭕ Malignancy

- ⭕ Recent Surgery
- ⭕ Birth Control Pills
- ⭕ Hormone Therapy

- ⭕ Previous Mapping
- ⭕ Obesity
- ⭕ Anticoagulation

- ⭕ Pregnancy
- ⭕ Varicose Veins
- ⭕ Polycythemia

Hyper-coagulability State:_____

Study: ⭕ Right ⭕ Left ⭕ Bilateral

Preliminary Impression

Right _____

_____

_____

_____

_____

Left _____

_____

_____

_____

_____

Thrombus:
⭕ Acute   ⭕ Chronic   ⭕ Recanalization

Preliminary Report As Requested
Review By _____ Time _____
Phoned to _____ Time _____

	IVC/ Iliac	CFV R/L	PFV R/L	SFV R/L	Pop R/L	PTV R/L	Saph R/L
Compressible							
Spontaneous							
Phasic							
Augment							
Partial Comp							
Partial Flow							

Figure 6.2 Deep vein thrombosis worksheet.

LE Venous Duplex for Reflux

Examination

Lower Extremity Venous Duplex for Reflux

Purpose

To evaluate the deep and superficial venous systems for evidence of valvular incompetence

Equipment Utilized

- Duplex Ultrasound machine with Spectral Doppler, Color Doppler and B-mode capabilities
- 5-12 MHz linear probe

Patient Preparation and Positioning

- Introduction to patient and a brief explanation of the examination
- Obtain pertinent patient history
- Brief examination of the lower extremities for signs of venous insufficiency- varicose veins, stasis changes, ulcers
- Patient puts on shorts or drape to allow for examination of entire leg
- Patient is placed in a standing position with the leg to be examined slightly externally rotated and weight on the contralateral limb

Examination Technique

- Study may be unilateral or bilateral
- Equipment gain and display settings should be optimized to provide the best possible B-mode images; color flow Doppler is utilized to assist in identifying vessels
- Spectral waveforms are obtained using a Doppler angle of sixty degrees or less, keeping the cursor aligned parallel to the vessel wall
- Distal compression of the limb is used to test for reflux
- Transverse probe compression maneuvers are performed every 2 cm along entire vein to test for DVT
- The entire lower extremity venous system should be assessed using both imaging and Doppler interrogation, obtaining hardcopy documentation as required by the Documentation Acquisition portion of this protocol

Documentation Acquisition

The following documentation must be obtained with additional documentation of questionable and abnormal or incidental findings.

- B-mode images of <u>diameter measurements</u> (transverse):
  - GSV at the saphenofemoral junction
  - GSV at mid thigh (zone 3)
  - GSV at knee (zone 5)
  - GSV at mid calf (zone 7)
  - SSV at the saphenopopliteal junction or popliteal fossa
  - SSV at mid calf (zone 7)
- B-mode images with <u>probe compression maneuvers every 2 cm</u> using split screen (transverse):
  - CFV
  - SFJ
  - GSV at mid thigh (zone 3)
  - GSV at knee (zone 5)
  - GSV at mid calf (zone 7)
  - Mid FV
  - Pop V
  - SSV at the saphenopopliteal junction or popliteal fossa
  - SSV at mid calf (zone 7)
  - Inferior Vena Cava (IVC), Common Iliac Vein (CIV), External Iliac Vein (EIV), Proximal FV, calf veins, and perforating veins are documented when necessary

Figure 6.3 Venous insufficiency evaluation protocol.

LE Venous Duplex for Reflux

- Spectral Doppler waveforms with <u>distal compression of the limb</u> (longitudinal):
  - ‣ CFV
  - ‣ SFJ
  - ‣ GSV at mid thigh (zone 3)
  - ‣ GSV at knee (zone 5)
  - ‣ GSV at mid calf (zone 7)
  - ‣ FV

  - ‣ Pop V
  - ‣ SSV at the saphenopopliteal junction or popliteal fossa
  - ‣ SSV at mid calf (zone 7)
  - ‣ Areas of suspected reflux
  - ‣ IVC, CIV, EIV, Proximal FV, calf veins, perforating veins and other accessory venous tributaries are documented when necessary
- Record all findings on the technologist's worksheet.

Special Considerations

- For obese patients, it may be necessary to use a lower frequency transducer
- For patients that have open draining ulcers, it may be necessary to use a probe cover
- Patients with severe edema that can impede accurate assessment of the calf vessels
- Patients who are unable to stand for an extended period of time that can impede accurate assessment of reflux

Reviewed

Date: _____ Medical Director: _____ Technical Director: _____

Figure 6.3 *(Continued)* Venous insufficiency evaluation protocol.

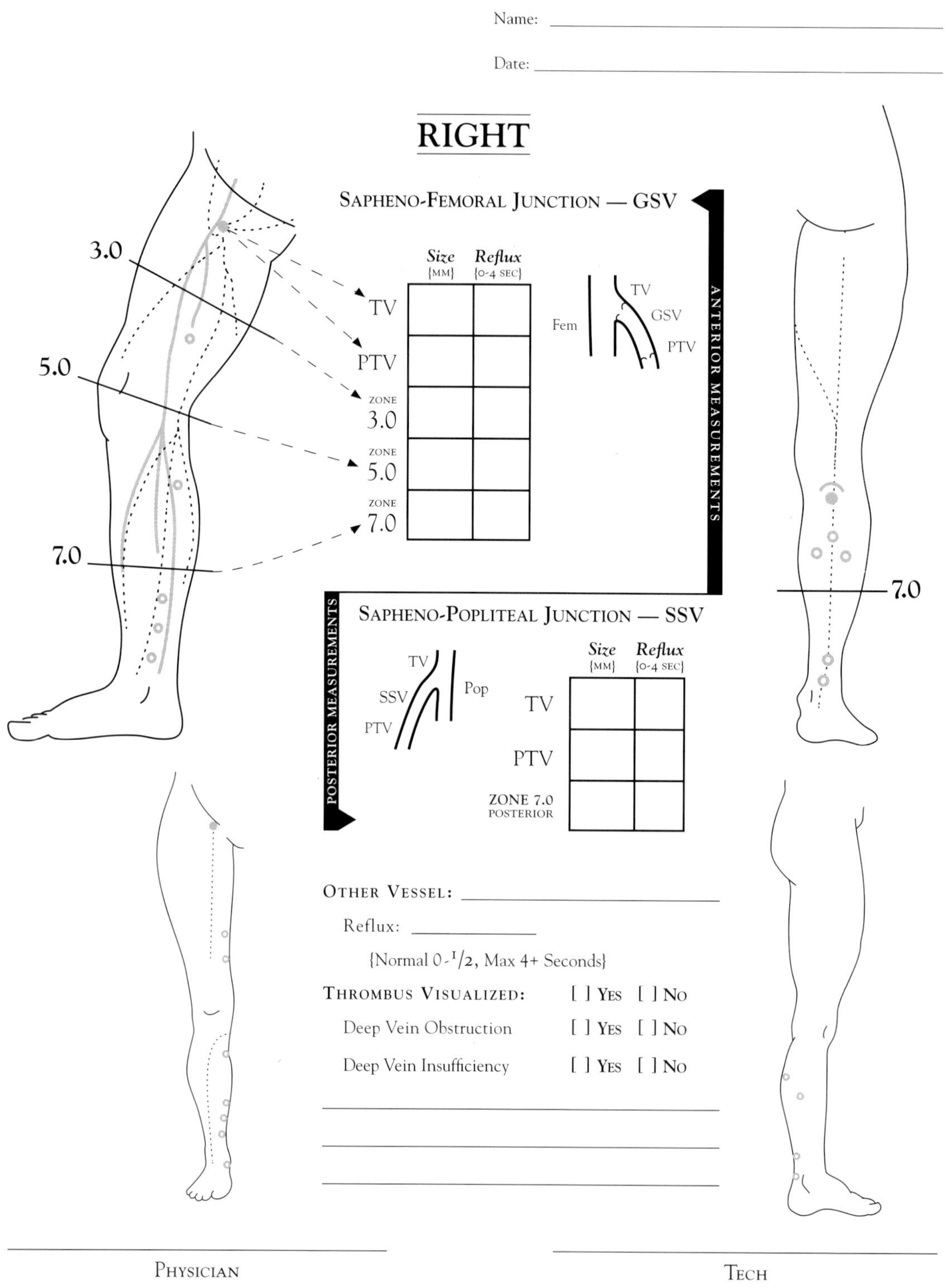

Name: _____

Date: _____

RIGHT

SAPHENO-FEMORAL JUNCTION — GSV

3.0

5.0

7.0

ANTERIOR MEASUREMENTS

	Size {MM}	Reflux {0-4 SEC}
TV		
PTV		
ZONE 3.0		
ZONE 5.0		
ZONE 7.0		

TV
Fem GSV
PTV

7.0

POSTERIOR MEASUREMENTS

SAPHENO-POPLITEAL JUNCTION — SSV

TV
SSV Pop
PTV

	Size {MM}	Reflux {0-4 SEC}
TV		
PTV		
ZONE 7.0 POSTERIOR		

OTHER VESSEL: _____

Reflux: _____

{Normal 0-$^{1}/_{2}$, Max 4+ Seconds}

THROMBUS VISUALIZED: [ ] YES   [ ] NO

Deep Vein Obstruction   [ ] YES   [ ] NO

Deep Vein Insufficiency   [ ] YES   [ ] NO

_____
_____
_____

_____
PHYSICIAN

_____
TECH

Figure 6.4 Venous insufficiency worksheet (one page for the right leg and one page for the left leg).

Figure 6.4 *(Continued)* Venous insufficiency worksheet (one page for the right leg and one page for the left leg).

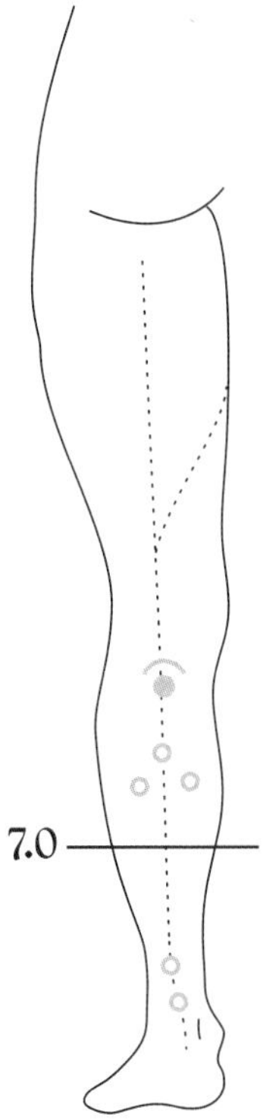

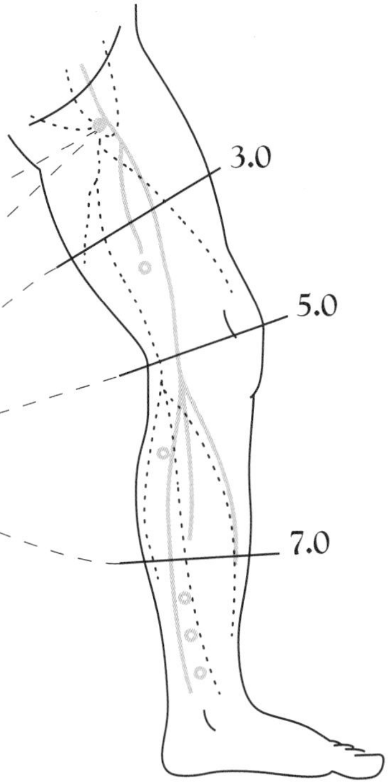

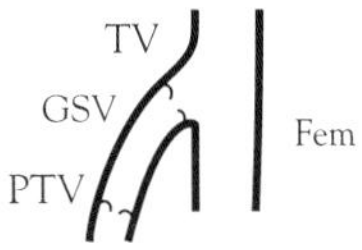

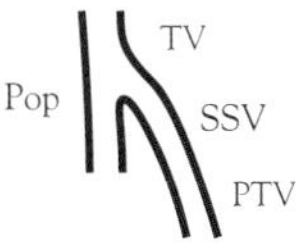

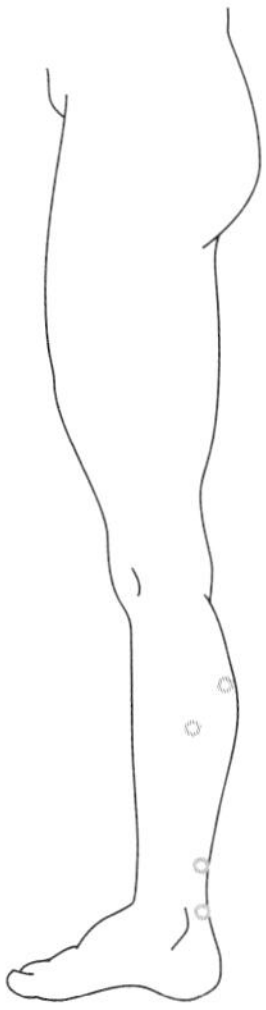

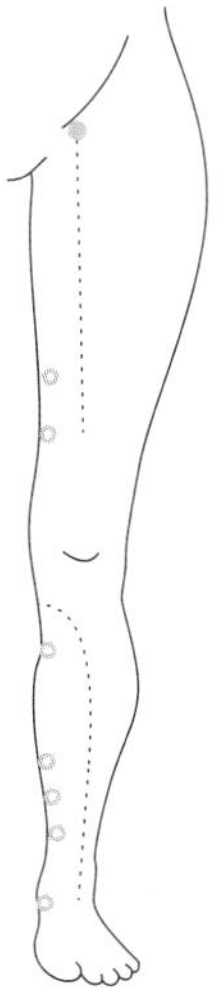

knowledge required for all sonography professionals and students. The specialty examinations include some physics and instrumentation content, and questions that are unique to that specialty.

The Vascular Technology specialty examination is 3 hours long and contains approximately 170 multiple-choice questions. These questions are related to disease states and performance and knowledge of testing findings.

Content outlines for both examinations are available on the ARDMS website and may change periodically. Information provided should be considered a starting point and contact made directly with that organization for the most up to date information.

Prerequisites

The ARDMS currently offers nine prerequisites (pathways) under which to apply for an ARDMS examination. An applicant must select a prerequisite under which he or she wants to apply for an ARDMS specialty examination and/or the SPI examination.

Each prerequisite requires (1) the appropriate educational background, (2) necessary clinical ultrasound or vascular experience, and (3) required documentation that must be submitted with the application. All three components of the prerequisite applied for must be met before an application can be approved and an applicant can be allowed to sit the examination (Figures 6.5 and 6.6).

To maintain an active ARDMS status you must (1) earn a minimum of 30 ARDMS-accepted continuing medical education (CME) credits in your three-year CME period and (2) pay an annual membership/renewal fees. There are discussions of a ten-year period with retesting, but this has not been currently adopted.

Registered Vascular Specialist

Cardiovascular Credentialing International is a not-for-profit corporation established in September 1988, for the sole purpose of administering credentialing examinations as an independent credentialing agency. CCI was formed following the merger of the testing components of the National Alliance of Cardiovascular Technologists (NACT),

the American Cardiology Technologists Association (ACTA), and the National Board of Cardiovascular Testing (NBCVT). CCI represents the summation of testing processes for the cardiovascular professional that began in the 1960s. There are currently approximately 2200 registered vascular specialists (RVS). Contact details: www.cci-online.org; 1500 Sunday Drive, Suite 102, Raleigh, NC 27607, USA; Telephone: 001 919 861 4539 or 001 800 326 0268.

In July 2010, CCI changed their testing procedures. To earn the RVS credential, applicants are now required to pass a one-part examination process. Although this is a one-part process, the examination contains knowledge-based questions from the information that was previously contained in two separate parts.

Examination qualifications

All applicants must meet the following criteria: (1) have a high school diploma or general education diploma at the time of application, (2) fulfill one of the five qualifications of the examination for which you are applying (see Figure 6.7), and (3) provide typed documentation to support the qualification under which you are applying.

CCI registrants keep their credentials up to date through a three-part process: (1) the submission of triennial (three-year) renewal fees, (2) signature and submission of a code of ethics statement, and (3) the accrual of 36 continuing educational units (CEUs) on a triennial basis.

New CCI registry credential in phlebology

In April 2010, CCI released a new venous-only vascular ultrasound credential, that of the registered phlebology sonographer (RPhS). The focus of this credential is venous disease and chronic venous insufficiency. The requirement for this credential grew out of the significant increase in interest in phlebology-based procedures and the diagnostic testing that accompanies this field. As of November 2012, the following are statistics about the RPhS examination:

Number of applicants taking the examination, 182

Examination Prerequisite Chart

The Sonography Principles and Instrumentation (SPI) Examination Requirement may be found on page 14.

Prerequisite requirements are subject to change at any time and from time to time. Applicants must meet current prerequisite requirements in effect at the time of application.

Prerequisite **1**

Education
A single two-year allied health education program that is patient-care related[1]

Allied health occupations include, but are not limited to, diagnostic medical sonographer, radiologic technologist, respiratory therapist, occupational therapist, physical therapist and registered nurse.

+

Required Clinical Ultrasound/Vascular Experience
12 months of full-time[2] clinical ultrasound/vascular experience [3]

Note: If you are using your DMS program for the educational requirement, you still have to document an **additional** 12 months of clinical ultrasound/vascular experience earned outside the two-year program.

+

Documentation Required with Application
1) Official transcript from two-year allied health education program is noted under the above "Education" requirement. Must state specific number of credits and indicate quarter or semester based system
and
2) Copy of education program certificate, credential or license
and
3) Original letter from supervising physician, sonographer/technologist or educational program director indicating a minimum of 12 months of full-time clinical/vascular experience including exact dates of ultrasound experience/ successful completion of sonography program as shown on page 15
and
4) Original signed and completed clinical verification (CV) form for each appropriate specialty area(s). **CV forms are located on pages 31-35.**

Prerequisite **2**

Education
Graduate of a program accredited by an agency recognized by the Council for Higher Education Accreditation (CHEA), United States Department of Education (USDOE) or Canadian Medical Association (CMA), that specifically conducts programmatic accreditation for diagnostic medical sonography/diagnostic cardiac sonography/vascular technology.

Required Clinical Ultrasound/Vascular Experience
No additional experience is required.

Documentation Required with Application
1) Copy of diploma from ultrasound/vascular program or an official transcript indicating the date the degree was conferred
and
2) Original letter signed by program director and/or medical director indicating date of graduation or successful completion of the program[4]. Program directors must use the mandatory formatted sample letter, available at www.ARDMS.org/PDletter.pdf, as shown on page 16
and
3) The CV form is not required if the application is submitted and received in the ARDMS office within one year after successful completion of the program. Otherwise an original signed and completed CV form for each appropriate specialty area(s) must be submitted. **CV forms are located on pages 31-35.**

Prerequisite **3A**

Education
Bachelor's degree (any major) or foreign degree equivalent to a Bachelor's degree in the U.S. or Canada

+

Required Clinical Ultrasound/Vascular Experience
12 months of full-time [2] clinical ultrasound/vascular experience [3]

+

Documentation Required with Application
1) Copy of Bachelor's degree or an official transcript earned in the U.S. or Canada or an original foreign transcript evaluation indicating that the degree is equivalent to a Bachelor's degree in the U.S. or Canada
and
2) Original letter from supervising physician, sonographer/technologist or educational program director indicating a minimum of 12 months of full-time clinical/vascular experience including exact dates of ultrasound experience/ successful completion of sonography program shown on page 15
and
3) Original signed and completed clinical verification (CV) form for each appropriate specialty area(s). **CV forms are located on pages 31-35.**

Figure 6.5 American Registry for Diagnostic Medical Sonographers prerequisite chart (multiple pathways exist).

Prerequisite
3B

Education

Bachelor's degree in sonography or vascular technology or foreign degree equivalent to a Bachelor's degree in sonography or vascular technology in the U.S. or Canada.

+

Required Clinical Ultrasound/Vascular Experience

No additional experience is required.

Note: Sonography or vascular technology Bachelor's degree applicants may take the examination one year prior to the completion of degree, provided they have completed 12 months of full-time clinical experience within the program.

+

Documentation Required with Application

1) Copy of Bachelor's degree or an official transcript earned in the U.S. or Canada or an original foreign transcript evaluation indicating that the degree is equivalent to a Bachelor's degree in the U.S. or Canada
and
2) Original letter signed by education program director verifying length of ultrasound or vascular experience. If program is not completed at the time of application a letter signed by the program director stating graduation date and completion of appropriate clinical ultrasound experience [3] is needed [5]. Program directors must use the mandatory formatted sample letter, available at www.ARDMS.org/PDletter.pdf, as shown on page 16
and
3) The CV form is not required if the application is submitted and received in the ARDMS office within one year prior to successful completion of the program, provided that the applicant has completed 12 months of full-time clinical experience within the program at the time that the application is submitted. Otherwise an original signed and completed clinical verification (CV) form for each appropriate specialty area(s) must be submitted. **CV forms are located on pages 31-35.**

Prerequisite
4A1

Education

General, U.S., and Canada — MD or DO degree earned in the U.S. or Canada
and
Formal Training — Attendance of an Accreditation Council for Graduate Medical Education (ACGME) or Royal College of Physicians and Surgeons of Canada (RCPSC) accredited residency or fellowship that includes didactic and clinical ultrasound/vascular experience as an integral part of the program.

+

Required Clinical Ultrasound/Vascular Experience

The applicant must be able to document clinical experience with a minimum of 800 studies in the area in which he/she is are applying for.

+

Documentation Required with Application

1) Copy of medical school diploma
and
2) Original letter from residency/fellowship program director verifying dates of attendance and completion of a minimum of 800 studies in the area in which you are applying
and
3) Original signed and completed clinical verification (CV) form for each appropriate specialty area(s). CV forms are located on pages 31-35.
and
4) Applicants should maintain a patient log or other record of the 800 studies. This log does not need to be submitted with the application but may be requested as part of a random audit. This documentation should be maintained by the application for at least three (3) years following the date of application for examination.

Prerequisite
4A2

Education

General, U.S., and Canada — MD or DO degree earned in the U.S. or Canada

+

Required Clinical Ultrasound/Vascular Experience

12 months of full-time clinical ultrasound/vascular experience.

+

Documentation Required with Application

1) Copy of medical school diploma
and
2) Original letter from supervising physician, sonographer/technologist or educational program director indicating a minimum of 12 months of full-time clinical/vascular experience including exact dates of ultrasound experience/successful completion of sonography program (visit www.ARDMS.org/sampleletters for examples). If you are the supervising physician, you may write your own letter.
and
3) Original signed and completed clinical verification (CV) form for each appropriate specialty area(s). CV forms may be found at: www.ARDMS.org/CV. CV forms are located on pages 31-35.

Prerequisite
4B1

Education

General — Outside U.S. — MD or DO degrees equivalent to those of the U.S. or Canada
and
Formal Training — Attendance of an accredited residency or fellowship that includes didactic and clinical ultrasound/vascular experience as an integral part of the program.

+

Required Clinical Ultrasound/Vascular Experience

The applicant must be able to document clinical experience with a minimum of 800 studies in the area in which he/she is are applying for.

+

Documentation Required with Application

1) Original credential report or official notarized copy of the evaluation converting the foreign medical degree must indicate that this medical degree is equivalent to a doctor of medicine degree in the U.S. or Canada. A listing of organizations that produce individualized, written reports describing each certificate, diploma or degree earned, and specifying its U.S. or Canadian equivalent can be found at www.ARDMS.org/ForeignTranscripts. If the applicant has taken and passed all three parts of and earned the Educational Commission for Foreign Medical Graduates (ECFMG®) certification, a copy of the ECFMG® certificate may be submitted with a copy of a current, valid MD or DO license from the U.S. or Canada in lieu of the evaluation.
and
2) Original letter from residency/fellowship program director verifying dates of attendance and completion of a minimum of 800 studies in the area in which you are applying
and
3) Original signed and completed clinical verification (CV) form for each appropriate specialty area(s). CV forms are located on pages 31-35.
and
4) Applicants should maintain a patient log or other record of the 800 studies. This log does not need to be submitted with the application but may be requested as part of a random audit. This documentation should be maintained by the application for at least three (3) years following the date of application for examination.

Figure 6.5 *(Continued)* American Registry for Diagnostic Medical Sonographers prerequisite chart (multiple pathways exist).

Prerequisite
4B2

Education

General — Outside U.S. — MD or DO degrees equivalent to those of the U.S. or Canada

+

Required Clinical Ultrasound/Vascular Experience

12 months of full-time clinical ultrasound/vascular experience.

+

Documentation Required with Application

1) Original credential report or official notarized copy of the evaluation converting the foreign medical degree must indicate that this medical degree is equivalent to a doctor of medicine degree in the U.S. or Canada. A listing of organizations that produce individualized, written reports describing each certificate, diploma or degree earned, and specifying its U.S. or Canadian equivalent can be found at www.ARDMS.org/ForeignTranscripts. If the applicant has taken and passed all three parts of and earned the Educational Commission for Foreign Medical Graduates (ECFMG®) certification, a copy of the ECFMG® certificate may be submitted with a copy of a current, valid MD or DO license from the U.S. or Canada in lieu of the evaluation.

and

2) Original letter from supervising physician, sonographer/technologist or educational program director indicating a minimum of 12 months of full-time clinical/vascular experience including exact dates of ultrasound experience/successful completion of sonography program (visit www.ARDMS.org/sampleletters for examples). If you are the supervising physician, you may write your own letter.

and

3) Original signed and completed clinical verification (CV) form for each appropriate specialty area(s). CV forms are located on pages 31-35.

Prerequisite
5

Education

General — Must hold an Active certification with Cardiovascular Credentialing International (CCI)-RCS or RVS, American Registry of Radiologic Technologist (ARRT)-Vascular Sonography, Sonography or Breast, or Australian Society of Ultrasound in Medicine (ASUM)-DMU.

+

Required Clinical Ultrasound/Vascular Experience

Previously met by achievement of other organization's credential.

+

Documentation Required with Application

1) Copy of Active certification identification card or copy of license

and

2) Original signed and completed CV form for each appropriate specialty area(s). CV forms are located on pages 31-35.

ARDMS offers an Application Submission Checklist towards the end of this application. Please remove this checklist and use it to ensure you submit all the necessary documentation with your application. You can also obtain additional copies of the ARDMS Application Submission Checklist by visiting www.ARDMS.org/checklist.

Figure 6.5 *(Continued)* American Registry for Diagnostic Medical Sonographers prerequisite chart (multiple pathways exist).

ARDMS®
The globally recognized standard of excellence in sonography

Standard Clinical Verification Form
(For the AB, OB/GYN, NE, VT, AE and PE exams)

All of the Clinical Verification Forms (Standard, Breast, Fetal Echocardiography and International) are available online by visiting www.ARDMS.org/cv. **You must use a separate form for each applied-for specialty examination.** Please submit this form with your completed application.

Applicant's Name: _____ Applied-for Specialty: _____(only one)
Applicant's ARDMS number (if applicable): _____

To be eligible to sit for all specialty examinations, the applicant must be able to consistently demonstrate the following minimum core clinical skills necessary to establish eligibility for ARDMS examinations. Applicants are responsible for meeting the requirements at the time of application.

Clinical Verification	Sponsor's Initials (Sign for Each Section)
1. Interact appropriately with the patient, physicians and staff.	
2. Identify the pertinent clinical questions and the goal of the examination.	
3. Recognize significant clinical information and historical facts from the patient and the medical records, which may impact the diagnostic examination.	
4. Review data from current and previous examinations to produce a written/oral summary of technical findings, including relevant interval changes, for the interpreting physician's reference.	
5. Select the correct transducer type and frequency for examination(s) being performed.	
6. Adjust instrument controls including examination presets, scale size, focal zone(s), overall gain, time gain compensation, and frame rate to optimize image quality.	
7. Demonstrate knowledge and understanding of doppler ultrasound principles, spectral analysis, and color flow imaging relevant to specialty being assessed.	
8. Demonstrate knowledge and understanding of anatomy, physiology, pathology and pathophysiology relevant to specialty being assessed.	
9. Demonstrate the ability to perform sonographic examinations of the appropriate organs and areas of interest according to professional and employing institution protocols.	
10. Recognize, identify and document the abnormal sonographic patterns of disease processes, pathology, and pathophysiology of the organs and areas of interest. Modify the scanning protocol based on the sonographic findings and the differential diagnosis.	
11. Perform related measurements from sonographic images or data.	
12. Utilize appropriate examination recording devices to obtain pertinent documentation of examination findings.	

Note: This form is valid for one year from the signature date of the Sponsor. This form must be signed by someone who is ARDMS Registered in the applied-for specialty area. This form must contain original (signed) initials and signatures. Original initials must be included for each numbered skill, above. Facsimiles and photocopies of signatures or initials are not acceptable. ARDMS conducts random audits of some applications for examination. Applicants who are audited will be required to submit additional documentation to substantiate eligibility.

Sponsoring Sonographer Verification Statement:
My signature verifies I am currently ARDMS-registered in the _____ Specialty requested by this applicant. This applicant has successfully demonstrated entry-level clinical skills as listed on the Clinical Verification Form for _____ Specialty.

I understand submitting false documentation to ARDMS is a violation of ARDMS rules and may result in sanctions including but not limited to revocation of my certification and eligibility for registration in all categories, including those already held.

I, _____, sponsoring sonographer, of _____, certify that the applicant named hereon has completed the minimum core procedures necessary to establish eligibility acceptance for the ARDMS Specialty Sonography Examination.

_____   _____   _____
Signature of Sponsoring Sonographer   ARDMS number   Date (MM/DD/YYYY)

_____   _____
Name (Please Print)   Business Phone

Figure 6.6 American Registry for Diagnostic Medical Sonographers clinical verification form.

Registered Vascular Specialist (RVS)

Qualification Requirements

All applicants must meet the following criteria:

1. Have a high school diploma or general education diploma at the time of application.

2. Fulfill one (1) of the qualifications of the exam for which you are applying. See qualifications listed in the tables below.

3. Provide typed documentation to support the qualification under which you are applying. Required documentation for each qualification is listed below. CCI reserves the right to request additional information.

Qualification Prerequisite #	Qualification Prerequisite	Supporting Documentation
RVS1	Two (2) years (full-time or full-time equivalent) in Vascular Ultrasound at the time of application.	Employment Verification Letter
RVS2	An Associate Degree or equivalent college hours (62 semester hours) in health, science, natural science, nursing, engineering, or any primary science and one (1) year (full-time or full-time equivalent) in Vascular Ultrasound at the time of application.	Completion certificate and/or educational transcript AND Employment Verification Letter
RVS3	A baccalaureate degree in health, science, natural science, nursing, engineering, or any primary science and six (6) months (full-time or full-time equivalent) in Vascular Ultrasound at the time of application.	Completion certificate and/or educational transcript AND Employment Verification Letter
RVS4	A graduate of an accredited program in Vascular Sonography (Vascular Ultrasound). **	Completion certificate and/or educational transcript AND Student Verification Letter
RVS5	A graduate of a NON-programmatically accredited program in Vascular Sonography (Vascular Ultrasound) which has a minimum of one (1) year of specialty training and includes a minimum of 800 clinical hours in the specialty in which the examination is being requested.	Completion certificate and/or educational transcript AND Student Verification Letter AND Clinical Verification Letter*

* **IMPORTANT**: If an individual's clinical hours were obtained after graduation or if the hours are not a requirement for their educational program, then those hours WOULD NOT count toward the 800-hour minimum under qualification RVS5.

** An accredited program is accredited by an agency recognized by the Council for Higher Education Accreditation (CHEA), United States Department of Education (USDOE), or Canadian Medical Association (CMA) that specifically conducts <u>programmatic</u> accreditation for cardiovascular technology, diagnostic cardiac sonography, or vascular technology.

The current examination qualifications are presently due to be updated effective **July 1, 2013**. Applicants applying on or after **July 1, 2013** will be required to meet the updated qualification criteria. Please refer to CCI's web site or contact CCI Headquarters for additional information.

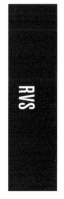

Figure 6.7 Registered Vascular Specialist (Cardiovascular Credentialing International's prerequisite chart).

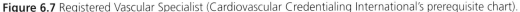

Number of applicants who have passed the examination, 120

Number of physicians who passed, 20

Number of sonographers who passed, 100

The RPhS examination was recognized by the LCD (local coverage determination) L29234 (Medicare guidelines) for the state of Florida for reimbursement, as noted in the excerpt from the document below.[8] The LCD for Tennessee and Puerto Rico were revised to include the RPhS.

Additionally, the IAC (Intersocietal Accreditation Commission) is considering recognition of this credential, as well as the creation of a new Phlebology Facility credential.

- Examples of certification in vascular technology for non-physician personnel include:
  - Registered vascular technologist credential
  - Registered vascular specialist credential
  - Registered phlebology sonographer
- These credentials must be provided by nationally recognized credentialing organizations, such as:

- The American Registry of Diagnostic Medical Sonographers which provides credentials for diagnostic medical sonographers and registered vascular technologists
- The Cardiovascular Credentialing International which provides credentials for registered vascular specialists and registered phlebology sonographers
- Appropriate nationally recognized laboratory accreditation bodies include: Intersocietal Commission for the Accreditation of Vascular Laboratories (ICAVL) and the College of Radiology (ACR).

The RPhS has its own application process with prerequisites for both sonographer (non-physicians) and physicians as noted in Figure 6.8.

Scope of practice note

As a side but related note, CCI also has a credential for invasive cardiovascular pesonnel who participate in catheterization laboratory procedures. The scope of practice for the registered cardiovascular invasive specialist (RCIS) is significantly different than that for the classic sonographer. People not familiar with the scope of practice are advised to download 'scope of practice' documents from SMDS, SVU and AIUM with regard to sonographer limitations. See Figure 9.2 on page 162. For instance, the state of Florida's Medicare LCD also has specific language preventing a sonography technician from 'administration of therapy'. These documents, including those by CCI for the invasive cardiovascular professional, can be examined online. Local or state variances can also vary as recently pointed out in Indiana with regard to the invasive cardiovascular professional which specifically states that sonographers may not 'administer medication' unless otherwise licenced to do so.

Accreditation

Laboratory accreditation in vascular ultrasound is available from two main organizations: the ICAVL (a division of the IAC) and the ACR.

Currently, laboratory accreditation in vascular ultrasound is voluntary but many insurance carriers, including Medicare, require that vascular studies be performed by credentialed vascular technologists or in accredited vascular laboratories in order to receive reimbursement. The policy changes and updates happen frequently and the best source of information is the insurance carrier or Medicare itself. Provided here is a link to the Medicare LCD policy page on the internet to investigate this issue on a state by state basis with the most up-to-date information that is available (www.cms.gov/mcd/index_lmrp_bystate_criteria.asp?from2=index_lmrp_bystate_criteria.asp&).

Intersocietal Commission for the Accreditation of Vascular Laboratories

ICAVL, a non-profit organization, was incorporated in 1990 in response to the need for standardization and improvement of the quality of non-invasive vascular laboratories. This was the first of the now six divisions that function under the umbrella of the IAC. Although the IAC accredits other imaging specialties, the focus below will be the vascular division, historically known as ICAVL. The purpose of the ICAVL is 'to ensure high quality patient care and to promote health care by providing a mechanism to encourage and recognize the provision of quality non-invasive vascular diagnostic testing by a process of voluntary accreditation'. The ICAVL website provides a wealth of information on the accreditation process. Contact information: www.intersocietal.org/vascular 6021 University Boulevard, Suite 500, Ellicott City, MD 21043, USA; Telephone: 001 800 838 2110.

ICAVL accreditation is currently offered in the following testing areas: (1) extracranial cerebrovascular, (2) intracranial cerebrovascular, (3) peripheral arterial, (4) peripheral venous, (5) visceral vascular, and (6) screening. A practice can apply for accreditation in any combination of the above areas of testing. Peripheral venous testing would be the appropriate testing area to be accredited for a phlebology practice. According to ICAVL, the number of sites looking for venous-only accreditation has increased significantly over the past few years (Katanick, personal communication).

ICAVL has 'standards' for performing and reporting ultrasound studies. These include: Part I,

Registered Phlebology Sonographer (RPhS)

Qualification Requirements

All applicants must meet the following criteria:

1. Have a high school diploma or general education diploma at the time of application.

2. Fulfill one (1) of the qualifications of the exam for which you are applying. See qualifications listed in the tables below.

3. Provide typed documentation to support the qualification under which you are applying. Required documentation for each qualification is listed below. CCI reserves the right to request additional information.

Qualifications: Non Physician Applicants

Qualification Prerequisite #	Qualification Prerequisite	Supporting Documentation
RPhS1	Hold an active RVS or RVT credential plus six (6) months (full-time or full-time equivalent) of diagnostic ultrasound experience in venous disease at the time of application. **AND** 36 CMEs in last four (4) years documented in venous disease, ultrasound diagnosis, or vascular anatomy.	Employment Verification Letter (from a supervising physician or credentialed lab director) **AND** verification of status as "ACTIVE" from appropriate credentialing agency (example: copy of registrant card) **AND** CME Documentation (See page 62 for required format)
RPhS2	An associate degree or equivalent college hours (62 semester hours) in health, science, natural science, nursing, engineering, or any primary science and one (1) year (full-time or full-time equivalent) diagnostic ultrasound experience in venous disease. **AND** 36 CMEs in last four (4) years documented in venous disease, ultrasound diagnosis, or vascular anatomy	Completion certificate and/or educational transcripts **AND** Employment Verification Letter **AND** CME Documentation (See page 62 for required format)
RPhS3	A baccalaureate degree in health, science, natural science, nursing, engineering, or any primary science and six (6) months (full-time or full-time equivalent) of diagnostic ultrasound experience in venous disease at the time of application. **AND** 36 CMEs in last four (4) years documented in venous disease, ultrasound diagnosis, or vascular anatomy	Completion certificate and/or educational transcripts **AND** Employment Verification Letter **AND** CME Documentation (See page 62 for required format)
RPhS4	Two years (full-time or full-time equivalent) experience in diagnostic ultrasound in venous disease at the time of application. **AND** 36 CMEs in last four (4) years documented in venous disease, ultrasound diagnosis, or vascular anatomy	Employment Verification Letter **AND** CME Documentation (See page 62 for required format)

The current examination qualifications are presently due to be updated effective **July 1, 2013**. Applicants applying on or after **July 1, 2013** will be required to meet the updated qualification criteria. Please refer to CCI's web site or contact CCI Headquarters for additional information.

Figure 6.8 Registered Phlebology Sonographer application prerequisites.

Registered Phlebology Sonographer (RPhS)

Qualifications: Physician Applicants

Qualification Prerequisite #	Qualification Prerequisite	Supporting Documentation
RPhS5	Valid license to practice medicine at the time of application AND Holds certification through the American Board of Phlebology or holds an active RVS, RVT, or RPVI credential AND Diagnostic ultrasound experience in venous disease indicated by performing or directly supervising a minimum of 150 venous studies within the two years prior to the application.	Copy of Medical License AND Verification of status as "ACTIVE" from appropriate credentialing agency (example-copy of registrant card) AND Notarized letter from a supervising physician, credentialed lab director, or office manager that verifies the number of venous studies performed or directly supervised and the period of time during which the studies were performed. (Physicians in solo practices may sign off on their letter.)
RPhS6	Valid license to practice medicine at the time of application AND Diagnostic ultrasound experience in venous disease indicated by performing or directly supervising a minimum of 200 venous studies within the two years prior to the application.	Copy of Medical License AND Notarized letter from a supervising physician, credentialed lab director, or office manager that verifies the number of venous studies performed or directly supervised and the period of time during which the studies were performed. (Physicians in solo practices may sign off on their letter.)
RPhS7	Valid license to practice medicine at the time of application AND Completion of a residency or fellowship that includes specialized clinical training in phlebology ultrasound performance and interpretation. Performing or directly supervising venous ultrasound studies, a minimum of 200 obtained during the training program.	Copy of Medical License AND Completion certificate and/or educational transcripts AND Notarized letter from program director/supervisor that verifies the program's length, the number of studies and the period during which the studies were performed.

The current examination qualifications are presently due to be updated effective **July 1, 2013**. Applicants applying on or after **July 1, 2013** will be required to meet the updated qualification criteria. Please refer to CCI's web site or contact CCI Headquarters for additional information.

Figure 6.8 *(Continued)* Registered Phlebology Sonographer application prerequisites.

Organization and Part II, Vascular Laboratory Operations. The standards are extensive documents that define the minimal requirements for non-invasive vascular laboratories to provide high quality care and must be used when preparing for accreditation.

Part I, Organization, is required for all of the testing areas. The organization standard takes a look at the supervision and personnel in the laboratory and their credentials, what support services are provided to ensure safe and efficient patient care, how the physical facility is set up, information about the examination interpretation, final report, and record keeping, as well as patient safety, confidentiality, and quality assurance/quality control issues.

Part II, Vascular Laboratory Operations, is specific to the testing area. For the purpose of this manual,

we concentrate on peripheral venous testing. This standard takes a look at the instrumentation used, the indications for testing, techniques, and documentation of examination performance, as well as diagnostic criteria and interpretation, procedure volumes, and quality assurance.

Additional requirements when applying for accreditation include the submission of case studies, the number of which is determined by several factors which are described in the application process. Also the laboratory could potentially be required to undergo a site visit by ICAVL. This could be either a random or required site visit which is scheduled at a time that is agreed upon by the laboratory and ICAVL.

Once the laboratory receives accreditation, it is valid for three years and then must be renewed.

American College of Radiology

The American College of Radiology, with more than 30 000 members, is the principal organization of radiologists, radiation oncologists, and clinical medical physicists in the United States. The college is a non-profit professional society whose primary purposes are to advance the science of radiology, improve radiologic services to the patient, study the socioeconomic aspects of the practice of radiology, and encourage continuing education for radiologists, radiation oncologists, medical physicists, and people practicing in allied professional fields. Contact information: www.acr.org; 1891 Preston White Drive, Reston, VA 20191, USA; Telephone: 001 800 770 0145.

The ACR has accredited approximately 10 000 practices and 20 000 facilities. The very first radiographic technician registered by the ACR was Sister M Beatrice Merrigan, in November 1922.

The Ultrasound Accreditation Program involves the acquisition of clinical images, submission of relevant physician reports corresponding to clinical images submitted, and quality control documentation. This is another pathway for laboratory accreditation for radiology practices. The ACR's accreditation program office is also available by phone listed above.

REFERENCES

1. ACR Practice Guideline for Performing and Interpreting Diagnostic Ultrasound Examinations – revised, 2010. Available from: www.acr.org. Last accessed December 10, 2010.
2. Lurie F, Comerota A, Eklof B *et al*. Multicenter assessment of venous reflux by duplex ultrasound. *Journal of Vascular Surgery* 2012; **55**: 437–45.
3. Baker S, Willey B, Mitchell C. The attempt to standardize technical and analytic competence in sonography education. *Journal of Diagnostic Medical Sonography* 2011; **27**: 203–11.
4. American Registry for Diagnostic Medical Sonography (ARDMS) website. Available from: www.ardms.org. Last accessed December 20, 2010.
5. ICAVL standards for accreditation in non-invasive vascular testing – 4/10. Available from: www.icavl.org. Last accessed April 15, 2010.
6. Society of Vascular Ultrasound Professional Performance Guidelines. Lower extremity venous insufficiency evaluation. Available from: www.svunet.org.
7. Veinz, Inc. Phlebology consulting services. Venous insufficiency worksheets, 10.09.
8. Medicare First Coast Options LCD 29234. Available from: http://medicare.fcso.com. Last accessed February 9, 2011.

7

Pre-, intra-, and post-treatment use of duplex ultrasound

Introduction

The advent of venous duplex ultrasound opened our eyes to understanding of the anatomy and pathology of the venous system. Furthermore, it assisted further in the evaluation of the outcomes of interventions, which were relatively poor with previous approaches to saphenous stripping. With increased understanding of the reasons for failures and advancing thought, duplex greatly influenced the manner in which we currently approach venous disease, leading to the development of endovenous techniques as first described in 2001.[1–3] As applied in today's therapeutic environment, duplex ultrasound has three distinct roles: pretreatment evaluation, intraoperative guidance, and post-therapy evaluation, and continues to add to advancing thought. The UIP (Union Internationale de Phlébologie) consensus document on the post-treatment evaluation brings several key points to light regarding sonography and vein therapy, and should be required reading.[4]

Pretreatment duplex evaluation

Chapter 6 described protocols and elements of a venous duplex examination. Paramount in this process is the patient's presenting condition and tailoring the duplex examination with the goal of understanding the pathology. For successful treatment to occur, accurate diagnosis and directed treatment is critical. It is not unreasonable to understand that failure to identify and treat all sources of reflux will lead to early recurrence. As noted in the vein map in Figure 7.1a, it is easy to understand that the anterior accessory great saphenous vein (AAGSV) is refluxing, while the proximal great saphenous vein (GSV) is not refluxing. This finding is also demonstrated in the corresponding duplex image Figure 7.1b, which shows refluxing color flow in the AAGSV, and not in the GSV or femoral vein. The duplex image alone indicates the origin of the reflux, but not the path. The addition of the vein map demonstrates much more fully the course of the reflux, and would allow for a more tailored approach to be undertaken.

Creation of a vein map which demonstrates the anatomy and refluxing patterns has become a standard process in most vein clinics. Drawing a vein map may seem daunting to beginners, and a step-by-step process is described later in this chapter. For the novice, beginning with a basic and simple map focusing on the GSV in the thigh can be a good starting place. Figure 7.1c shows this basic approach. Approximately 70 percent of patients have reflux in the GSV, so it should be recognized that this basic map would only meet the need of seven out of ten patients. As skills develop with the map creation technique, a more detailed map will seem less daunting.

As noted in the UIP consensus document, 'the morphology and hemodynamic abnormalities relating to varices and location should be noted on a diagram. … an exhaustive report with a diagram is suggested.'[5] The process of taking B-mode images and transferring them to a vein map can be perceived to be a challenging task. Described below are key elements for this process.

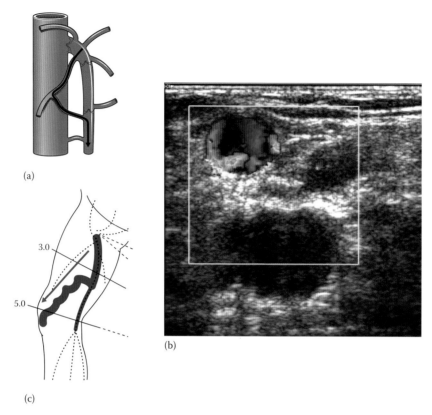

(a)

(b)

(c)

Figure 7.1 (a) Vein map diagram showing reflux down an accessory vein, without reflux in the proximal great saphenous vein (GSV). Lower down, the path of reflux re-enters the GSV proper. (b) In the ultrasound image, reflux is noted in the dilated anterior accessory great saphenous vein, and not in the GSV or common femoral vein. (c) Basic vein map showing reflux from the SFJ down the GSV to a large anterior tributary at mid thigh.

One key consideration in creating a vein map is to focus on providing information that will assist in treatment planning. Vein mapping always starts with the foundation (the saphenous compartment) and the vein(s) within it. In Figure 7.2a, the GSV is identified in the saphenous sheath while, with color flow Doppler, the refluxing varicose vein is noted above the fascia in the epifascial space. The key point would be to trace the saphenous vein, determine if there is a connection with the refluxing varicose vein, and 'source' the reflux back to its probable saphenous origin. As noted in Figure 7.2b, there can be a network of varicose veins noted which could be confusing at first glance. In this instance, tracing out the veins will allow the saphenous vein to be identified within the sheath, while the varices will be above the compartment in the epifascial area. Generally speaking, most of all pathology will have involvement of the saphenous vein with extensions from the saphenous to more superficial varicosities.

Working in this fashion from the saphenous compartment up to the surface varices is very helpful for the novice.

Creating a vein map – step-wise process

Once you have progressed past the basic vein map concept as noted above, a more advanced mapping process will reveal and document more information that will be invaluable for the treatment process. When scanning any saphenous vein, focus first only on the saphenous vein in its compartment. Realize that several diameter measurements are required along the course of the vein, and this is the first clue to pathology. A simple example of how to draw a vein map is broken down here going from ultrasound image to vein map. A saphenous vein that changes size dramatically is an indication of

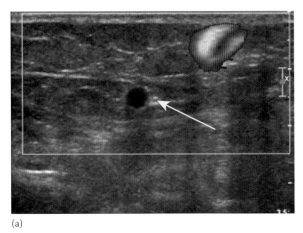

(a)

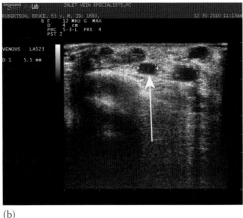

(b)

Figure 7.2 (a) The saphenous vein is easily noted in the compartment, without reflux, and the refluxing superficial varicose vein is colorized in the epifascial space. (b) This image depicts a network of varicosities in close proximity to the great saphenous vein which could be confusing to the novice. By tracing this out, and looking at the compartment, the true saphenous vein can be identified (within the compartment) as compared to the varices seen above the compartment.

reflux entering or leaving the vein. Figure 7.3 shows the GSV (a) in the upper thigh and (b) at the knee. Note how there is a significant change in the diameter of the GSV. This indicates that reflux has left the compartment, since the GSV is smaller.

By slowly tracing the GSV from the area where Figure 7.3a was taken and Figure 7.3b was taken, a large tributary vein is noted, with a corresponding decrease in size of the GSV distal to the tributary. Looking at Figure 7.4, a thicker GSV proximal, a large tributary coming off, and a thinner GSV below the tributary are shown.

A question often asked is, 'Do I have to draw out all branches and tributaries that I see during the ultrasound on the vein map?' As a general rule of thumb, only those tributaries 50 percent or greater in size, as compared to the GSV, need to be indicated on the vein map. The exception to this would be if a varicose complex is traced or sourced back to a saphenous vein. In this instance, the tributary needs to be indicated regardless of size.

To make this task less daunting, a step-by-step process will be suggested as describe below.

Break the saphenous investigation process into four parts: (1) the small saphenous below the popliteal fossa, (2) the cranial extension of the small saphenous, (3) the great saphenous in the thigh (adding the anterior accessory great saphenous vein as needed), and (4) the great saphenous in the leg. By using a step-by-step process, a vein map

can be completed in segments as noted in Figure 7.5a–d.

The diagram or worksheet is critical in this process. On the sample provided in Chapter 6, note that the 'normal' location of the deep system is noted as gray lines, while the saphenous and its major tributaries are drawn as dotted lines (as a guide for location purposes) and when mapping drawn on the form. Other tips regarding the use of this form include:

1) There are boxes for the measurement of the great saphenous vein at the junction (terminal valve (TV), and preterminal valve (PTV)), the mid-thigh (zone 3.0), knee (zone 5.0), and mid-calf (zone 7.0). These zones are only points of reference, with zone 1.0 being in the inguinal crease and 9.0 being the ankle level. Most protocols suggest that multiple saphenous vein diameters be documented.

2) These boxes also allow for documentation of reflux at each level. Reflux should be noted in time intervals, i.e. 0.5 or 2+ seconds, and not simply positive or negative (+/−), also ***avoid the terms 'mild, moderate, or severe' as these subjective and not standardized.***

3) For the small saphenous, proximal measurements (near the TV and/or PTV) and the mid-calf (zone 7.0) on the posterior aspect are noted.

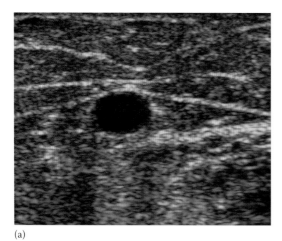

(a)

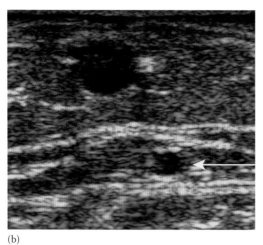

(b)

Figure 7.3 (a) Larger great saphenous vein (GSV) in the sheath; (b) smaller GSV in the sheath (arrow) and the larger tributary.

4) The open circles indicate typical location of perforating veins. Please note that the posterior tibial perforators are not along the GSV, but the posterior arch vein (posterior accessory saphenous of the leg).
5) There is a section for indicating 'other vessel' findings, such as AAGSV.
6) There are areas to indicate the presence of absence of thrombus, and deep vein obstruction or insufficiency, which can be checked for normal, but it is suggested that more detail be provided for any pathologic findings.
7) A 'Notes' section (several blank lines) is provided to further extrapolate upon anything of interest. Depth of the vein when less than 1 cm should be noted here,

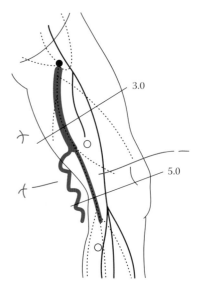

Figure 7.4 Vein diagram of the great saphenous vein and a large medial distal tributary (thigh).

especially if endovenous thermal ablation is a consideration, and for access site planning. Adding information regarding any large straight refluxing vein which is suprafascial is also helpful.
8) There are also lines for both the person performing the scan (technologist) and the interpreting physician to sign.
9) Reflux can be denoted with a colored pen (in our office, a blue line or a (+) symbol indicated reflux. Other methods include the use of arrows to indicate the direction of flow along the vein.

There exist several versions of worksheets or documentation methods, any of which can be used, as long as all the appropriate diagnostic information is provided. Keep in mind that the worksheet is to facilitate the gathering of information, and not limit it. The samples provided have undergone multiple revisions over the past 15–20 years, adapting to the evolving field of phlebology and the treatment techniques at our disposal.

Below are vein map diagrams (Figure 7.6) showing several different patterns of reflux and pathology. Visualizing these various diagrams supports the need to understand the pattern of pathology in planning intervention. Several more vein maps are provided in Chapter 8 for additional reference.

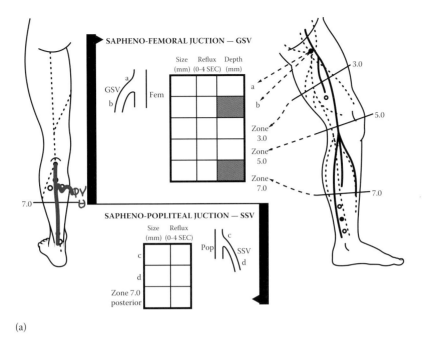

(a)

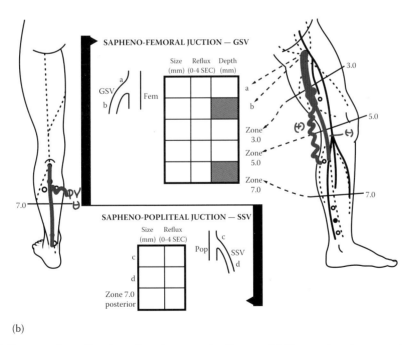

(b)

Figure 7.5 (a) The posterior calf and small saphenous vein diagram. (b) The great saphenous vein (GSV) in the thigh is added next. (c) The GSV in the leg is detailed. (d) Vein size and other details are added to the vein map.

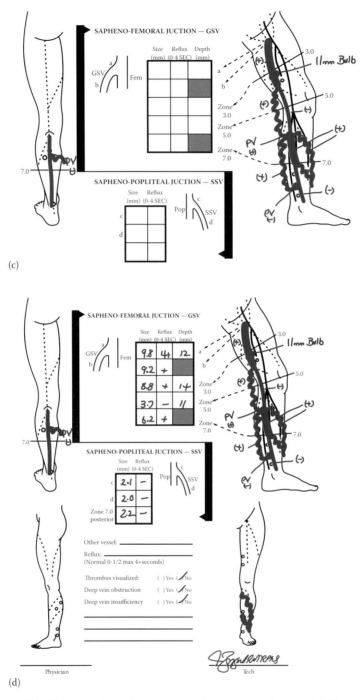

Figure 7.5 *(Continued)* (a) The posterior calf and small saphenous vein diagram. (b) The great saphenous vein (GSV) in the thigh is added next. (c) The GSV in the leg is detailed. (d) Vein size and other details are added to the vein map.

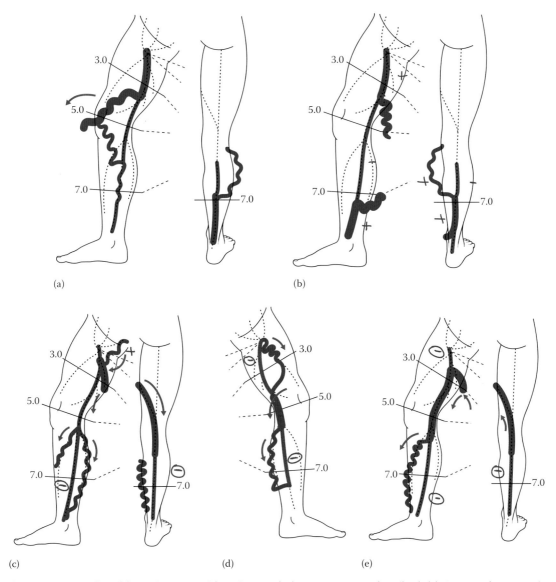

Figure 7.6 Examples of five vein maps with various pathology patterns as described. (a) Great saphenous vein (GSV) with reflux in large anterior tributary that circles laterally and connects to small saphenous vein at mid-calf. (b) GSV with reflux into large median tributary descending along medial calf. (c) Normal saphenofemoral junction, reflux from pudendal source into GSV below junction with distal saphenous varicose complex. (d) Anterior saphenous reflux down thigh, connecting to GSV at knee with reflux into posterior arch vein in distal leg. (e) Flow from saphenopopliteal junction ascending in cranial extension leading to reflux down the GSV from about zone 3, with distal anterior tibial varices.

Intraoperative duplex applications

The addition of duplex ultrasound to guide therapeutic intervention adds to the accuracy but also the safety of the procedures undertaken. This application is being used in many fields of medicine for biopsy, nerve blocks, regional anesthesia, insertion of catheters and central lines to name but a few. In the following pages, discussion points will focus upon concepts related to ablation procedures, specifically: (1) preoperative marking; (2) access for intervention; (3) placement and advancement (or positioning) of the catheter; (4) administration of tumescent anesthesia; (5) monitoring treatment, and (6) immediate post-treatment imaging.

Preoperative marking

Immediately prior to an ablation procedure, a preoperative scan is typically performed, during which preoperative marking is completed. This step clearly identifies the veins to be ablated. Scanning and tracing out the vein ensures understanding of anatomy, and any variables which will be encountered during the procedure, and is one of the most important steps to success. As noted in Figure 7.7, the course of the small saphenous vein (SSV) is marked out. A proximal mark indicates where the SSV dives to join the popliteal vein, and 5 cm hash marks along the course of the vein are placed to help estimate the approximate length of vein to be treated. As noted in Figure 7.8, the 20 cm mark lines up with a potential access site. For those physicians less comfortable with the procedure, or if the anatomy is challenging, the selection of two sites may be marked on the leg. Typically, a more distal access site is preferable, which allows as much of the refluxing vein to be ablated as possible. Note that these marks are placed on the leg prior to sterile preparation, with an indelible marker and serve as a guide during later aspects of the procedure. This

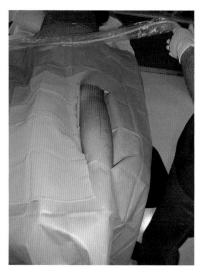

Figure 7.8 The posterior calf draped for the procedure showing the preoperative markings.

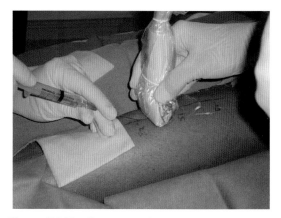

Figure 7.9 Needle access using a transverse approach. This shows the variation of using a syringe attached to the needle. Procedure images 7.7 to 7.9 courtsey Karl Hubach MD RVT RPhS.

same type of marking is performed for the GSV for identification of the saphenous junction.

Access

Access for ablation procedures is skillfully performed using ultrasound guidance. In Figure 7.9, a transverse approach is used for needle access. Note that in this instance, the physician has attached a syringe to the needle to aid in aspiration of blood to confirm placement. This step is not always done, however here the SSV was relatively small when

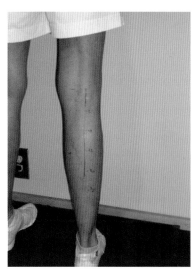

Figure 7.7 Preoperative marking of the course (and length) of the small saphenous vein.

decompressed in the prone position, and this technique can be very helpful. In larger veins, especially the GSV, an open needle technique is often used.

Ultrasound-guided needle access can be used in a variety of techniques including ultrasound-guided sclerotherapy with either a closed needle (syringe), open needle, or open or closed catheter techniques, including extended long line echosclerotherapy (ELLE), as described by Parsi.[6–8] Ultrasound-guided access is considered the standard approach for endovenous thermal ablation. There are two approaches to obtain venous access using ultrasound guidance: transverse and longitudinal. Using a simple phantom, these are demonstrated below. By using the probe

located over the vein, a puncture is made using either the long axis or short axis of the probe (Figure 7.10).

In Figure 7.11a,b, some of the difficulties are noted with relation to these approaches. In each approach, regardless of preference, a critical concept to understand is how the beam of ultrasound extends below the probe, and the width of the beam. In each of these images, note how the needle tip is well past the vein lumen.

Figure 7.12 illustrates the ultrasound beam as the 'speckled' area, and angulation and approach concepts are depicted.

Figure 7.13 using simply the probe and a needle further demonstrates the variations of trying to get the

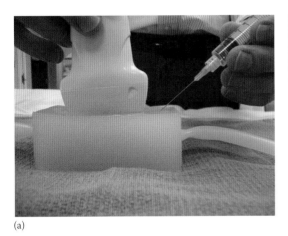

(a)

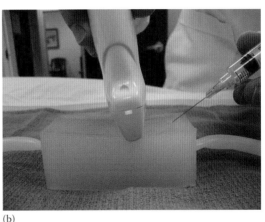

(b)

Figure 7.10 (a) Long axis and (b) short axis approach to vein access using a phantom.

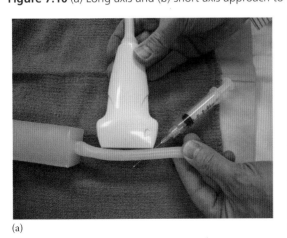

(a)

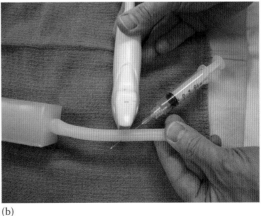

(b)

Figure 7.11 (a) This image shows the importance of knowing the exact position of the needle tip – in this instance below the vein and not in the lumen. Although the needle could be along the line of the ultrasound beam, the tip of the needle is not intravascular. (b) This image shows the difficulty in the transverse approach in which the needle is through the vein, however the needle tip is beyond the vein, and the ultrasound beam – and thus extravascular. Images courtesy Karl Hubach MD, RVT, RPhS.

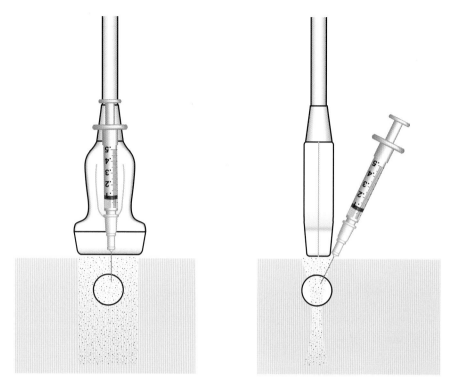

Figure 7.12 As shown here, the needle tip is intravascular – therefore using the correct angle and technique proves successful.

needle tip directly in the beam of the ultrasound so that the guided image is demonstrative of the process.

The transverse approach is widely used. A beginner's mindset is to realize that in the transverse approach, as the needle enters the field of view on the ultrasound monitor, it will appear as a bright white spot, as the needle 'pierces' the ultrasound beam. Using a relatively flat approach (needle flat to the skin approach), this white spot is noted in the near field. By using this indicator, the needle can be backed out of the field of view, while remaining in the skin, and the angle between the skin and the needle is increased (as noted in Figure 7.14) and the bright spot can be 'walked down' to the appropriate depth until the top of the vein wall tents. The long axis approach offers other advantages. In this scenario, the needle is 'driven' along the long axis of the probe. Done correctly, the needle will enter the ultrasound image and can be seen traveling along the image towards the vein until puncture is achieved. A key to success with this is in understanding that the ultrasound beam is very narrow, and proper alignment, as in the upper middle image of Figure 7.13, is critical.

Observation of the top wall of the vein proves to be a very reliable method to determine when the vein wall is actually pierced. As noted in Figure 7.15, due to the relatively lower pressure in a vein, it will often 'tent' until enough pressure is exerted to pierce the vein wall. This distortion of the vein wall is observed on the ultrasound monitor. In some cases, a double wall puncture is purposefully used and the needle is then slowly withdrawn, watching for the posterior wall to 'flop' off the needle to confirm positioning in the lumen.

Placement of the catheter

Ultrasound guidance is used not only for confirmation of the placement of the tip, but also can be used to assist in threading the catheter into the target vein. Figure 7.16 shows the short and long axis view of a radiofrequency catheter in a saphenous vein. The catheter is well visualized, and produces a shadow in the short axis image as noted. Another reason for a good preoperative scan is areas of slight tortuosity or passing through a bulbous dilation in the vein which can

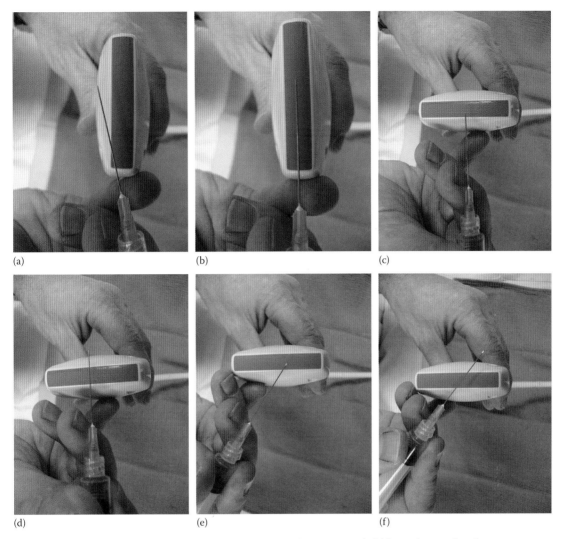

(a) (b) (c)
(d) (e) (f)

Figure 7.13 Using the probe and a needle, these photos demonstrate (a,b) how the needle alignment can be off, or appropriate, the needle tip may be (c) in the field or (d) past the field of view, and on an angle or oblique approach either (e) in the field, or (f) past the field of view of the ultrasound image. Images courtesy Karl Hubach MD, RVT, RPhS.

cause difficulty. Catheters can also become 'hung up' on valve cusps or other anatomic features. With the skillful use of ultrasound, the tip of the catheter can be visualized and the obstruction can be overcome with careful manipulation. Although a very tortuous vein cannot typically be threaded, with experience, a facile practitioner will be able to cannulate and treat somewhat more complex veins than the beginner. One should never advance a catheter forcefully against resistance otherwise vein perforation could occur.

Once the catheter is in the approximate location, perivenous anesthesia is applied to the saphenous compartment. During the application of perivenous anesthetic, the catheter could move, and therefore a conscientious practitioner will confirm tip placement immediately prior to perivenous anesthetic over the junctional area (if treating near the saphenofemoral junction (SFJ) or saphenopopliteal junction (SPJ)). Common practice is to measure a distance of 2+ cm from the SFJ. For the SPJ (SSV) observation of the fascial curve, as popularized by Elias, and (explained later in the text with other nerve considerations) for the proximal placement of the thermal catheter. Catheter tip placement can have a significant impact on endovenous heat-induced thrombus (EHIT)

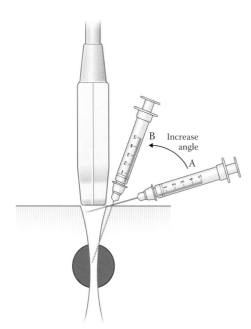

Figure 7.14 With the needle relatively flat to the skin (position A), the spot where the needle tip crosses the ultrasound beam is determined. Backing the needle out (without removing it from the skin) and increasing the angle to 'position B' and then, moving forward will result in the tip of the needle entering the plane of the ultrasound beam at a steeper and deeper level and, in this instance, actually closer to the vein.

tip measurement with calipers measuring this distance is strongly recommended as part of the medical record. A key aspect of this measurement is the size of the saphenous opening on the femoral vein,

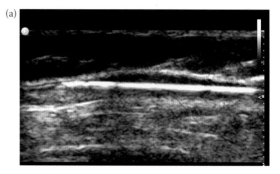

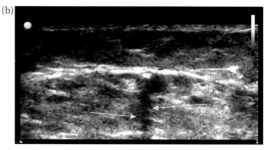

Figure 7.16 (a) ClosureFast™ Radiofrequency ablation catheter shown in the long axis, and (b) ClosureFast™ RFA catheter (red arrow) shown in the short axis with ultrasound shadow noted with yellow arrows. Images courtesy Antonio Gasparis, MD.

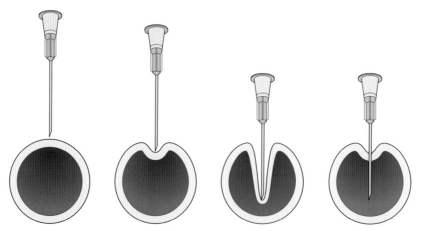

Figure 7.15 Vein 'tenting' with pressure, and in the image to the right, the needle finally pierces the vein wall.

extension,[9,10] also sometimes called post ablation superficial thrombus extension (PASTE) Figure 7.17 [1]

Although some practitioners omit this step, a digital frozen image with calipers showing the final and the impact this can have with regard to the point of measurement, i.e. the caliper placement.[12] In Figure 7.18, variations in the placement of the proximal caliper from the top of the femoral ova-

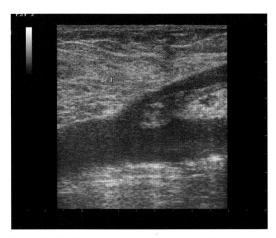

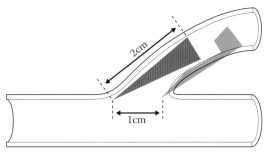

Figure 7.18 Variability in 2 cm measurement based on caliper placement (red, yellow, and green lights, similar to a traffic light representing stop, caution, and go).

Figure 7.17 Endovenous heat-induced thrombus extension at the saphenous junction.

lis to the bottom of that opening, can result in a significant variation on where the 2 cm measurement finally lands and the resulting proximity of the device to the femoral vein.

Once the final tip placement is confirmed, measured, and documented, additional perivenous tumescence is added at and above the junction. This step helps to ensure that the additional blood flow from the superior branches of the saphenous arch do not cause thermal cooling and less effective ablation of this area. Caution should be taken to avoid the femoral or other adjacent vessels to avoid injury, i.e causing a pseudoaneurysm or other complications.

Tumescent anesthesia for saphenous ablation

Duplex ultrasound guidance is invaluable for the application of anesthetic fluid to the saphenous compartment. The saphenous compartment, with its two fascial boundaries traps the perivenous anesthetic slowing down the dissipation of the fluid into surrounding tissues. The application of tumescent anesthetic accomplishes several things for a thermal ablation procedure: (1) This fluid creates a heat sink around the target vein, protecting surrounding tissues or if near the skin, can be used to 'push' the vein deeper away from the skin to prevent a burn. (2) The external compression exsanguinates the vein. (3) It compresses the vein closer to the heating element. Early experience with

thermal devices suggestsed that larger veins, or those with aneurysmal segments, may not be adequately treated with endovenous techniques. However, early adopters quickly learned the importance of skillful tumescent application, and 'very large' GSVs, up to 35 mm, have been ablated successfully with the radiofrequency (RF) procedure. It is apparent that well-placed anesthetic providing adequate external pressure on the vein constitutes an important factor in successfully treating venous (saphenous) incompetence with an ablation procedure.'[13]

As with needle access, perivenous anesthetic can be applied with either the transverse or the long axis approach with regard to the ultrasound guidance. This can be done with a syringe, or with a pump. Figure 7.19 shows application with a pump – note the tubing behind the physician's hand. If using a pump device, it is common to use the dark space created by the perivenous anesthetic as a target, and let the needle sit in that space while the pump 'hydrodissects' the saphenous compartment as the fluid surrounds the vein with increasing volume over a larger length Figure 7.20.

Another key application of duplex is appreciated more with higher resolution imaging systems which allow for clearer visualization of important nerves that are adjacent to the veins being treated. 'On transverse scans, the nerves appear as multiple round or oval hypoechoic areas encircled by a relatively hyperechoic horizon. The hyperechoic structures are the fascicles of the nerves, while the hypoechoic background reflects the connective tissue between the neuronal structures.'[14] The first paper using direct ultrasound (US) visualization for a regional anesthetic method (supraclavicular brachial plexus block) was published in 1994.[15]

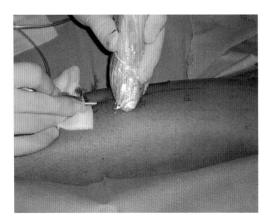

Figure 7.19 Perivenous anesthetic applied with a pump. Note tubing behind physician's hand.

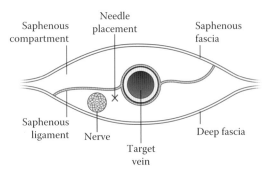

Figure 7.21 Separation of nerve from vein with directed needle approach for perivenous anesthetic can be achieved by those with increased skills.

With practice, nerves can be appreciated on duplex and application of perivenous anesthetic can be directed to 'push' a nerve further away from a vein, instead of perhaps closer towards it Figure 7.21.

There are four nerves that come into play most often with regards to phlebologic procedures, the saphenous nerve, the sural nerve, the tibial nerve, and the common peroneal nerve. The **saphenous nerve** is a sensory nerve relating to the medial calf, ankle, and foot. Murakami et al.[16] reported on the anatomical relationship of the saphenous vein and the saphenous nerve (Figure 7.22) indicating that these two ran intimately together in 59 percent in the middle third of the leg and 83 percent in the lower third of the leg. Additionally, more than half of those in the lower third of the leg showed

an 'adhesive relationship where the epineurium of the saphenous nerve was seen histologically to be attached to adventitia of vein'. Historically, with vein stripping, Masaki et al.[17] report that 4.9 percent of GSV strippings result in nerve injury and full length stripping accounted for almost 40 percent of all cases. Therefore, the relationship is well established, and should be recognized and safeguarded when using newer thermal approaches.

The **sural nerve** runs along the small saphenous vein in the mid-posterior calf and distally. It too is a sensory nerve, dealing with the lateral calf, ankle, foot, and calf. The sural nerve has been used in nerve transplantation cases. Furthermore, although a sensory nerve, it has been reported to have involvement with motor fibers in 4.5 percent of cases.[18] Reports from Proebstle et al.[19] and Gibson et al.[20] indicate sural neuropathy in 0–4.4 percent.

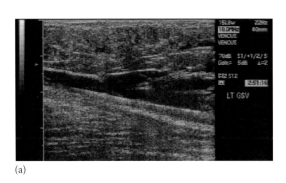

(a)

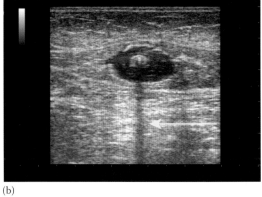

(b)

Figure 7.20 (a) Long axis or (b) short axis application of perivenous anesthetic anesthesia. Note in the short axis, the ultrasound shadow produced by the catheter.

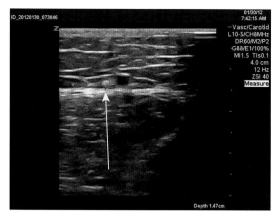

Figure 7.22 Duplex image of the saphenous vein and saphenous nerve (bright white to the left of the vein).

The **tibial nerve** is motor sensory in function. It lies in the popliteal fossa running alongside the popliteal artery (and other structures). Elias describes the 'fascial curve' as the area along the proximal small saphenous where the vein dives to meet the popliteal vein. This 'curve' is commonly used as a landmark in thermal ablation of the SSV, basically making sure the catheter tip does not extend into the dive or curve towards the popliteal vein (see figure 7.23 a,b). With injury to the tibial nerve, a patient will be unable to stand on tip toes, i.e. a loss of plantarflexion, and a sensory deficit on the sole of the foot. This nerve is historically thought of being at risk with trauma to the knee, or entrapment, but with aggressive manipulation or treatment in the popliteal fossa risks should be noted.

The **common peroneal nerve** also has a sensory–motor function (Figure 7.24 a,b). It is a distal branch of the sciatic nerve and can run along the lateral fibular head. Injury to the common peroneal nerve can result in foot drop with loss of sensation on the top of the foot. Incidence of injury with surgery to the small saphenous vein has been reported at 2–4.7 percent.[21] The relationship between the saphenopopliteal junction and the common peroneal nerve is well studied.[22] Due to the proximity of this nerve to the lateral fibular head, many practitioners use precautions with compression dressings or wraps so as to not cause entrapment and irritation of this nerve.

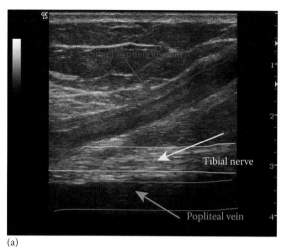

(a)

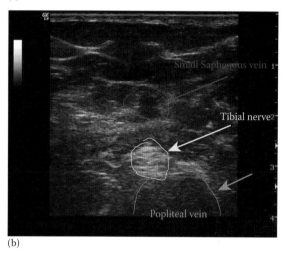

(b)

Figure 7.23 (a) Fascial curve. As the SSV dives, it approaches the popliteal vein. Note the orientation of SSV (red), hyperechoic tibial nerve (yellow) and popliteal vein (blue) in long view. (b) Orientation of SSV (red) as it approaches the junction with the popliteal vein. Note the proximity of the hyperechoic tibial nerve (yellow) and popliteal vein (blue) in this transverse view.

Duplex ultrasound monitoring during treatment

Monitoring the progress of treatment during thermal ablation is sometimes overlooked. However, this can add significant additional information to ensure safety during the procedure. First, the concept of ensuring that there is at least 1 cm of

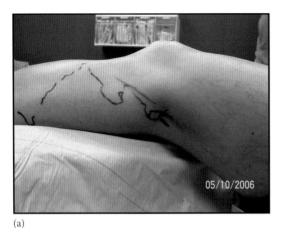

(a)

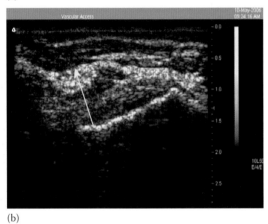

(b)

Figure 7.24 (a) Location of the common peroneal nerve along the lateral fibular head marked in red. The vein to be phlebectomized is marked in black. (b) Duplex image of the common peroneal nerve (indicated by yellow arrow).

distance between the thermal device and the skin surface is critical. If the perivenous anesthesia is around an epifascial vein, this fluid will dissipate into the surrounding tissues more quickly than if in the saphenous compartment, and thus monitoring this distance is strongly suggested. This is also a key step as one nears the insertion site, as the vein may be closer to the skin surface at this point.

Duplex is also helpful in observation of the vein during therapy. The 'action' that occurs near the tip provides confidence that the thermal generator, either RF or laser, is working properly and producing heat. Furthermore, observation of the location of the heating element can be followed. If the patient has an aneurysmal segment, extra thermal energy may be applied to that segment when it is

reached. This is also true for large side branches or perforators which can dump blood into the area and cause cooling. If duplex monitoring is not taking place, this could result in suboptimal treatment and potential early failure of one of these areas.

The specific location of the tip of the catheter (or heating element) can also be observed during treatment. Even with the safeguards that exist, there have been instances resulting in skin injury from thermal devices. An area of specific concern would also exist if treating the AAGSV. Due to this vein being located relatively closely and in 'alignment' with the femoral vein and artery, care needs to be taken to prevent injury to the deep vessels. There have been reports of an arteriovenous fistula being caused from laser energy being applied too close to arterial structures, one in the external iliac and one in the small saphenous region.[23, 24] Although in its own fascial sheath, Figure 7.25 demonstrates the proximity of an AAGSV to the femoral vessels. Extra care should be taken to thermally 'protect' the femoral vessels in situations such as these with adequate tumescence.

Our increased understanding of the importance of perivenous anesthesia is also in some fashion partly responsible for the technique of applying external compression over the thermal device during treatment. Many practitioners will use the duplex probe to apply direct pressure over the heating end of the catheter, monitoring the pullback under duplex to ensure compression over the segment of the vein being treated.

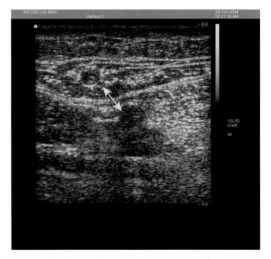

Figure 7.25 Anterior accessory great saphenous vein (AAGSV) post-ablation with femoral vessels in close proximity, as noted with the arrow.

The descriptions above relate mainly to thermal ablation. Nuances of each can equally be applied to any endovenous therapy, whether chemical, mechanical, or thermal. Some have even applied ultrasound guided tumescent anesthesia to greatly enhance traditional saphenous stripping.

The intraprocedural use of duplex has expanded our understanding of what is taking place during therapy. This is specifically in reference to the use of foam in sclerotherapy, and the migration of the foam bubbles. Morrison et al.[25] have contributed several publications to our understanding that all foam goes into the deep system, and circulates throughout the vasculature. Furthermore, Jia's group from the UK published an extensive review on this same issue.[26]

Duplex ultrasound following treatment

Following therapy, the use of duplex can be broken down into three separate and distinct applications: (1) immediate, (2) delayed, and (3) late interrogation. In addition to the immediate postoperative concern for deep vein thrombosis (DVT), these interrogations are performed for very similar reasons, and although the image characteristics and findings vary at each stage, we seek to ensure safety and verify outcome.

Immediate post-treatment interrogation has two main purposes. First, patency of the deep vein, either femoral (for GSV ablation) or popliteal (for SSV ablation) is confirmed with both Doppler and color flow analysis, and second the post-treatment vein wall and saphenous patency is examined. With regard to the deep system patency, the corresponding deep venous structures are examined for free flow and the lack of any thrombus. Also, and especially at the SFJ, patency and flow through the superficial epigastric vein (SEV) is also confirmed. This has two significant components. First, with maintainence of flow, the drainage of the abdominal wall or other pelvic sources is confirmed so 'frustrated drainage' which is hypothesized to cause neovascularization and a nesting of varices near the junction is avoided. Second, this flow from the SEV helps to 'wash out' the proximal GSV at the junction, helping to prevent the development of thrombus extension (EHIT). Figure 7.26 demonstrates all of these aspects.

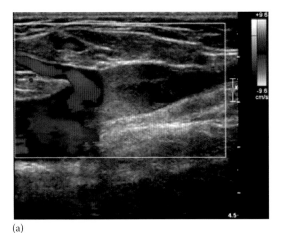

(a)

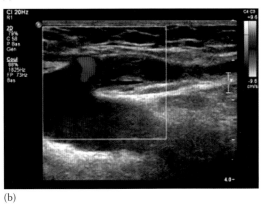

(b)

Figure 7.26 (a) Saphenofemoral junction (SFJ) immediately post-ablation with color flow in femoral and superficial epigastric vein, and no flow in the proximal great saphenous vein (GSV); (b) the SFJ 1 week post-treatment showing a reduction in the size of the diameter of the GSV.

The evaluation of the treated vein segment is also performed in the immediate post-treatment phase. Although the image quality is somewhat lessened following tumescence and treatment, the treated vein segment is evaluated. The vein should be smaller in diameter, showing evidence of inflammation and vein wall thickening. Sometimes, this is referred to as the 'donut' or 'cheerio' appearance of the vein wall (Figure 7.27). The vein itself does not necessarily have to have an obliterated lumen or a lumen with 'no flow' as the inflammatory changes progress or 'mature', resulting in a closed vessel.

During the delayed interrogation phase, a post-treatment evaluation is typically performed at an

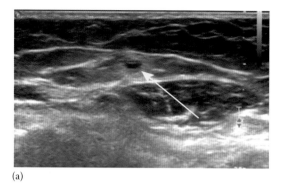

(a)

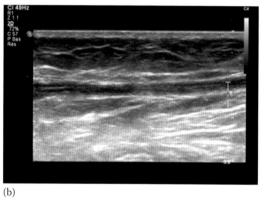

(b)

Figure 7.27 (a) In the transverse view, post-treatment, the great saphenous vein appears to be inflamed and thickened (like a cheerio), and (b) the same vein in a long axis view.

interval of 24–72 hours, although some wait up to a week for this examination. At this point, the basic findings desired are similar to those in the immediate post-treatment interrogation. Findings hope to confirm: (1) the absence of DVT; (2) flow in the SEV and the lack of thrombus extension (EHIT); and (3) lack of flow in the target vein with vein wall thickening and occlusion demonstrated. As described by Proebstle et al.,[27] 'substantial heat transfer to the vein wall leads to significant shrinkage of vein wall collagen fibers and consecutive reduction of the vein lumen. This fact is well known from radiofrequency closure …'. Proebstle et al. further state that 'the amount of vein wall shrinkage seems to be important because the remaining lumen of the vein … is subject to occlusion by endovascular clot formation …. Ideally, such a thrombotic occlusion … is replaced by a fibrotic cord that frequently can be detected even years after treatment.' The authors suggest further that this thrombotic occlusion is at risk to recanalization especially in larger veins. Pichot and his group[28] describe 'earlier stages in the maturing biologic process engendered by radiofrequency endovenous obliteration (RFO) are seen as a hyperechogenic strip with a narrow, contorted, echolucent lumen with no flow.' Furthermore, however, 'ultrasonic disappearance of the GSV trunk, as observed in 86 percent of the treated

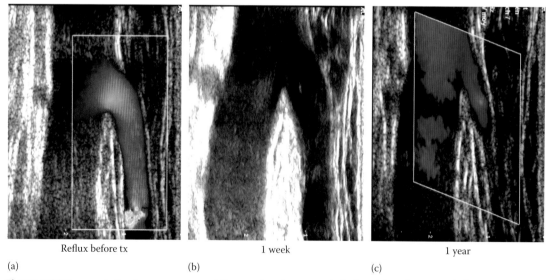

Reflux before tx   1 week   1 year

(a)   (b)   (c)

Figure 7.28 Demonstrates the appearance of the great saphenous vein before (a) and at 1 week (b) and one year (c) after radiofrequency treatment.

GSVs, marks complete vein wall involution.' The ultimate goal is the fibrotic, sclerotic process that takes many months to occur, resulting in the almost sonographically absent sclerotic cord that Pichot et al.[28] describe. Figure 7.28 demonstrates the appearance of the GSV before and after RF treatment. At 1 week follow up, the GSV trunk appears to be obliterated with an echoic lumen. At one year follow up, the GSV trunk appears to be shrunk with a small area of normal antegrade flow at the SFJ.

In conclusion, duplex ultrasound is an important tool for pretreatment evaluation, intraoperative guidance, and post-therapy evaluation and surveillance. Strongly recommended is additional reading of the paper cited at the opening of this section, that is the UIP consensus document on the post-treatment evaluation.[4]

REFERENCES

1. Navarro L, Min R, Bone C. Endovenous laser: a new minimally invasive method of treatment of varicose veins – Preliminary observations using an 810 nm diode laser. *Dermatologic Surgery* 2001; **27**: 117–22.
2. Min RH, Zimmet SE, Isaacs MN, Forrestal MD. Endovenous laser treatment of the incompetent greater saphenous vein. *Journal of Vascular Interventional Radiology* 2001; **12**: 1167–71.
3. Dauplaise T, Weiss RA. Duplex-guided endovascular occlusion of refluxing saphenous veins. *Journal of Vascular Techniques* 2001; **25**: 79–82.
4. De Maeseneer M, Pichot O, Cavezzi A *et al.* Duplex ultrasound investigation of the veins of the lower limbs after treatment for varicose veins – UIP Consensus Document. *European Journal of Vascular and Endovascular Surgery* 2001; **42**: 89–102.
5. Coleridge Smith P, Labropoulos N, Partsch H *et al.* Duplex ultrasound investigation of the veins in chronic venous disease of the lower limbs – UIP Consensus document. Part 1. Basic principles. *Phlebology* 2006; **21**: 158–67.
6. Parsi K, Lim AC. Extended long line echosclerotherapy. *Sclerotherapy Society of Australia News Bulletin* 1997; **1**: 10–12.
7. Min RJ, Navarro L. Transcatheter duplex ultrasound guided sclerotherapy for treatment of greater saphenous vein reflux: preliminary report. *Dermatologic Surgery* 2000; **26**: 410–14.
8. Parsi K, Lim AC. Extended long line echosclerotherapy. *Australia and New Zealand Journal of Phlebology* 2000; **4**: 6–10.
9. Kabnick L. New horizons of saphenous ablation. *Journal of Vascular Techniques* 2002; **26**: 239–46.
10. Dexter D, Kabnick L, Berland T *et al.* Complications of endovenous lasers. *Phlebology* 2012; **27**(Suppl. 1): 40–5.
11. Wright D, Morrison N, Recek C *et al.* Post ablation superficial thrombus extension (PASTE) into the common femoral vein as a consequence of endovenous ablation of the great saphenous vein. *Acta Phlebologica* 2010; **11**: 59–64.
12. Zygmunt J. Missed and mis-information on duplex. Presented at the American Venous Forum, Amelia Island, FL, February 2010.
13. Morrison N. VNUS closure of the saphenous vein. In: Bergan J (ed.). *The vein book*. Burlington, MA: Elsevier Press, 2007: 289.
14. Marhofer P, Greher M, Kapral S. Ultrasound guidance in regional anesthesia. *British Journal of Anesthesia* 2005; **94**: 7–17.
15. Kapral S, Krafft P, Eibenberger K *et al.* Ultrasound-guided supraclavicular approach for regional anesthesia of the brachial plexus. *Anesthesia and Analgesia* 1994; **78**: 507–13.
16. Murakami G, Negishi N, Tanaka K *et al.* Anatomical relationship between saphenous vein and cutaneous nerves. *Okajimas Folia Anatomica Japonica* 1994; **71**: 21–33.
17. Masaki K, Tetsuya N, Noriko N. Safety of outpatient vein stripping under local anesthesia and propofol sedation. *Japanese Journal of Phlebology* 2006; **17**: 11–16.
18. Nayak S. Sural nerve and short saphenous vein entrapment – a case report. *Indian Journal of Plastic Surgery* 2005; **38**: 171–2.
19. Proebstle TM, Gul D, Kargl A, Knop J. Endovenous laser treatment of the lesser saphenous vein with a 940-nm diode laser: early results. *Dermatologic Surgery* 2003; **29**: 357–61.
20. Gibson KD, Ferris BL, Polissar N *et al.* Endovenous laser treatment of the short saphenous vein: efficacy and complications. *Journal of Vascular Surgery* 2007; **45**: 795–803.

21. Atkin GK, Round VR, Vattipally VR, Das SK. Common peroneal nerve injury as a complication of short saphenous vein surgery. *Phlebology* 2007; **22**: 3–7.

22. Balasubramanian R, Rai R, Berridge DC *et al.* The relationship between the SPJ and the CPN: a cadaveric study. *Phlebology* 2009; **24**: 67–73.

23. Ziporin SJ, Ifune CK, MacConmara MP *et al.* A case of external iliac arterivenous fistula and high output cardiac failure after endovenous laser treatment of great saphenous vein. *Journal of Vascular Surgery* 2010; **51**: 715–19.

24. Timperman PE. Arteriovenous fistula after endovenous laser treatment of the short saphenous vein. *Journal of Vascular and Interventional Radiology* 2004; **15**: 625–7.

25. Morrison N, Neuhardt DL, Hansen K *et al.* Tracking foam to the heart and brain following ultrasound-guided sclerotherapy of lower extremity veins. *Australia and New Zealand Journal of Phlebology* 2007; **10**: 6–10.

26. Jia X, Mowatt G, Burr JM *et al.* Systematic review of foam sclerotherapy for varicose veins. *British Journal of Surgery* 2007; **94**: 925–36.

27. Proebstle T. Endovenous laser (EVL) for saphenous vein ablation. In: Bergan J (ed.). *The vein book.* Burlington, MA: Elsevier Press, 2007: 268.

28. Pichot O, Kabnick LS, Creton D *et al.* Duplex ultrasound scan findings two years after great saphenous vein radiofrequency endovenous obliteration. *Journal of Vascular Surgery* 2004; **39**: 189–95.

8

Forms and sample vein maps

Introduction

This chapter contains an example of a dictated duplex report, technical mapping worksheets for duplex studies, instructions for use, and completed versions of these worksheets with descriptions for each. The reader can use these worksheets as presented or alter to suit their needs. These are being presented as examples and suggestions of the type of information that could be presented in conjunction with venous duplex studies.

Venous duplex reporting

As noted in this chapter and elsewhere, upon completion of a duplex study, an 'official' interpretation needs to be created (typically dictated) by the interpreting physician (Figure 8.1). Current standards of care suggest that the duplex mapping form should accompany the official interpretation report to become a part of the final report and medical record.

Instructions for use: lower extremity venous duplex worksheet

This worksheet (Figure 8.2) is best used for evaluation of the deep system for obstruction – following the deep vein thrombosis (DVT) protocol. The vessels on the diagram indicate the deep veins of the lower extremities. As the 'instructions for use' document describes (Figure 8.3), other sections document pertinent information that should be collected for adequate presentation to the interpreting physician. One worksheet is adequate for a bilateral study as noted. Note: Occasionally, if DVT is found during a reflux exam for chronic venous insufficiency (CVI), this worksheet should be added to the system to fully document the deep venous findings.

Instructions for use: venous reflux worksheets

This worksheet is best used for the evaluation of patients with chronic venous insufficiency (varicose veins). The instructions for use (Figure 8.4) describe the information that could be gathered and presented. This worksheet has a right and left version, in order to present the nuances of venous pathways that develop in CVI patients (Figure 8.5a,b).

Following these blank versions, are several versions of each of the worksheets with examples of the findings that can be encountered in a practice dealing with CVI patients on a regular basis (Figures 8.6–8.19). These are presented for informational purposes to illustrate the versatility of the documents, and the types of information that can be presented to the interpreting physician regarding venous duplex examinations.

Report for Duplex Venous Ultrasound

Patient Name:
Date of Service:
Diagnosis: Chronic Venous Insufficiency, Sapheno-Femoral Junction Incompetence, Venous Varicosities, Leg Pain (459.89, 454.1)
Procedure: Duplex Ultrasound of the Deep and Superficial systems of the legs

Indication: chronic venous insufficiency, varicose veins, leg pain

LEFT LEG: Duplex imaging study was carried out according to normal protocol with the patient in a standing position. Imaging was performed with a 7.5Mhz imaging probe using B-Mode ultrasound. Deep veins were imaged from the level of the common femoral to the posterior tibial veins. All deep veins demonstrated compressibility without evidence of intraluminal thrombus or increased echogenecity. Doppler investigation was carried out with a 5.0Mhz pulsed gated crystal. Spectral analysis of Doppler signals demonstrates normal response to compression maneuvers indicating patency without obstruction. Reflux determinations were made with the patient in the standing position, the weight being on the contralateral leg.

The great saphenous vein system displayed compressibility without evidence of thrombophlebitis. The great saphenous vein measured **mm at the junction, mm at mid thigh, and mm at the knee, laying mm beneath the skin surface in the facial sheath.** Its terminal and subterminal valves (sapheno-femoral junction) displayed non-functioning venous valves, which resulted in 4+ seconds of reflux (retrograde blood flow) in this vein system. **The proximal great saphenous vein displays the absence of vein tortuosity severe enough to impede catheter placement or advancement, and without significant aneurismal dilation contraindicated in an ablation procedure.** Bulging **Two large bulbous dilatations are noted, one at mid thigh and one at the knee which measure and mm respectively.** A **large posterior branch floods reflux into the varicosities of the medial calf, and lower leg**. There are **two** incompetent perforating veins located **at the Boyd and Cockett's levels**. Each of these diseased veins dumps reflux into the varicose complex. This is a grossly convoluted varicose complex. The small saphenous vein measures mm at the sapheno-popliteal junction. It is normal with respect to size and hemodynamic function.

RIGHT LEG: Duplex imaging study was carried out according to normal protocol with the patient in a standing position. Imaging was performed with a 7.5Mhz imaging probe using B-Mode ultrasound. Deep veins were imaged from the level of the common femoral to the posterior tibial veins. All deep veins demonstrated compressibility without evidence of intraluminal thrombus or increased echogenecity. Doppler investigation was carried out with a 5.0Mhz pulsed gated crystal. Spectral analysis of Doppler signals demonstrates normal response to compression maneuvers indicating patency without obstruction. Reflux determinations were made with the patient in the standing position, the weight being on the contralateral leg.

The great saphenous vein system displayed compressibility without evidence of thrombophlebitis. The great saphenous vein measured **mm at the junction, mm at mid**

Figure 8.1 Sample duplex ultrasound report.

Report for Duplex Venous Ultrasound

thigh, and   mm at the knee, laying   mm beneath the skin surface in the facial sheath. Its terminal and subterminal valves (sapheno-femoral junction) displayed non-functioning venous valves, which resulted in 4+ seconds of reflux (retrograde blood flow) into this vein system. **The proximal great saphenous vein displays the absence of vein tortuosity severe enough to impede catheter placement or advancement, and without aneurismal dilation contraindicated to the procedure. Two large bulbous dilatations are noted, one at mid thigh and one at the knee which each measure   mm. A posterior branch floods reflux into the varicosities of the medial calf, and lower leg.** There are **two** incompetent perforating veins located **at the Boyd and Cockett's levels**. Each of these diseased veins dumps reflux into the varicose complex. The small saphenous vein measures **2-3** mm at the sapheno-popliteal junction. It is normal with respect to size and hemodynamic function.

IMPRESSION: Bilateral venous reflux from non-functioning venous valves is noted in the great saphenous and distal varicose veins. Dilated and **bulging** varicosities are noted bilaterally which are resultant from the **sapheno-femoral and perforating vein incompetence discussed above**. The deep venous system is within normal limits without evidence of obstruction or insufficiency.

John Doe MD, FACS, RPVI

NOTE: ITEMS IN YELLOW highlight MUST BE modified to the patient's specific pathology these statements are only examples to be modified as needed.

Other suggested Key Statements that may be included:
"duplex of lower extremities for chronic venous insufficiency"
"imaging performed with optimized settings using a variable frequency 7-10 MHz probe"
"doppler spectral analysis performed with optimized settings i.e. angles, gate etc using a 7.5MHz doppler crystal"
"deep system evaluation included coaptation of the following vessels to demonstrate patency and lack of obstruction" .....list vessels
"duration of reflux was ___seconds following release of distal compression using......."
"all reflux determinations were performed with the patient in the standing position"

Figure 8.1 (_Continued_) Sample duplex ultrasound report.

Lower Extremity Venous Duplex

Patient name: _____ Date: _____

Reffering M.D:_____ Study performed by: _____

Indications: _____ Prior Exam: Date/Result _____

History:

☐ Swelling   ☐ CHF   ☐ Recent Surgery   ☐ Previous Mapping   ☐ Pregnancy

☐ Smoking   ☐ Prior DVT   ☐ Birth Control Pill   ☐ Obesity   ☐ varicose veins

☐ Chemo/XRT   ☐ Malignancy   ☐ Hormone Therapy   ☐ Anticoagulation   ☐ Polycythemia

Hyper-coagulability State: _____

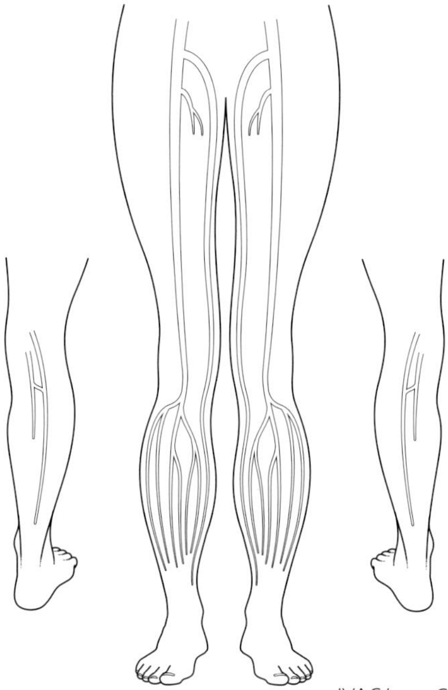

Study: ☐ Right ☐ Left ☐ Bilateral

Preliminary Impression

Right
_____
_____
_____
_____
_____

Left
_____
_____
_____
_____

Thrombus:

☐ Acute   ☐ Chronic   ☐ Recanalization

Preliminary Report As Requested

Reviewed by _____ Time _____

Phoned to _____ Time _____

	IVAC/ Iliac	CFV R/L	PFV R/L	SFV R/L	Pop R/L	PTV R/L	Saph R/L
Compressible							
Spontaneous							
Phasic							
Augment							
Partial Comp							
Partial Flow							

_____
Physician

_____
Tech

Figure 8.2 Deep vein thrombosis. Worksheet.

Instructions for Use
LE Venous Duplex Worksheet

This worksheet provides for gathering and documenting data obtained during an lower extremity venous ultrasound examination to rule out a deep venous thrombosis (DVT). This information can then be used to write/dictate a formal ultrasound report. This worksheet should remain as part of the patient's permanent record.

- The study can be either unilateral or bilateral but must follow the practices written protocol.

- Under 'Indications' choose symptoms/reasons that are appropriate for performing this study. Examples include- swelling, pain, superficial thrombophlebitis, etc.

- Use the table at the bottom of the form to document your findings.

- Then summarize your findings in the 'Preliminary Impression' section. These should be technical findings, not an interpretation of the results.

- If thrombus is found, be sure to categorize the thrombus as either acute, chronic or recanalized based on the criteria in your practices protocol.

- Depending on the practices protocol, a preliminary report should be made ASAP to the referring physician.

- The diagrams are available to document the extent of the thrombus.

Figure 8.3 Deep vein thrombosis. Instructions for use.

Instructions for Use
Venous Reflux Worksheets

These worksheets provide for gathering and documenting data obtained during a venous insufficiency ultrasound examination. This information can then be used to write/dictate a formal ultrasound report. These worksheets should remain as part of the patient's permanent record.

- The study can be either unilateral or bilateral but must follow the practices written protocol. There is a separate worksheet for each leg.

- Explanation of Diagrams:
  - The solid gray lines on the diagrams indicate the locations and path of the deep venous system.

  - The dotted black lines on the diagrams indicate the typical locations of the great and small saphenous veins along with major tributaries. These lines are dotted so that you can draw on the form either along the "normal" course of the vein, or to show an anatomical variation you may encounter during your mapping procedure.

  - The gray open circles on the diagrams indicate the typical locations of perforating veins.

  - The zones (3.0, 5.0, 7.0) are only points of reference, with zone 1.0 being in the inguinal crease and 8.0 being the ankle level. See the diagram titled "Zones for Ultrasound" for a full explanation.

- Explanation of sections:
  - The first section is for documentation of findings for the sapheno-femoral junction (SFJ) and great saphenous vein (GSV).

    - Great saphenous vein diameter measurements at the terminal valve (TV) and pre-terminal valve (PTV) of the sapheno-femoral junction (SFJ), the mid thigh (zone 3.0), knee (zone 5.0) and mid calf (zone 7.0).

    - There are also spaces for documentation of reflux at each level.

  - The second section is for documentation of findings for the sapheno-popliteal junction (SPJ) and small saphenous vein (SSV).

    - Small saphenous vein diameter measurements at the terminal valve (TV) junction (knee crease) and the mid calf (zone 7.0) on the posterior aspect are noted.

    - Cranial extension of the small saphenous vein (TH/EXT) and the vein of Giacomini (VOG) diameter measurements, if present.

    - There are also spaces for documentation of reflux at each level.

  - The third section is for documentation of "other vessel" findings as well as the presence of thrombus, deep venous obstruction and deep venous insufficiency. These can be checked for normal or abnormal, but it is suggested that more detail be provided for any pathologic findings.

  - The blank lines or "note" section is provided to further extrapolate upon anything of interest.

  - There are also lines for both the person performing the scan (tech) and the interpreting physician to sign.

Figure 8.4 Reflux worksheet: Instructions for use.

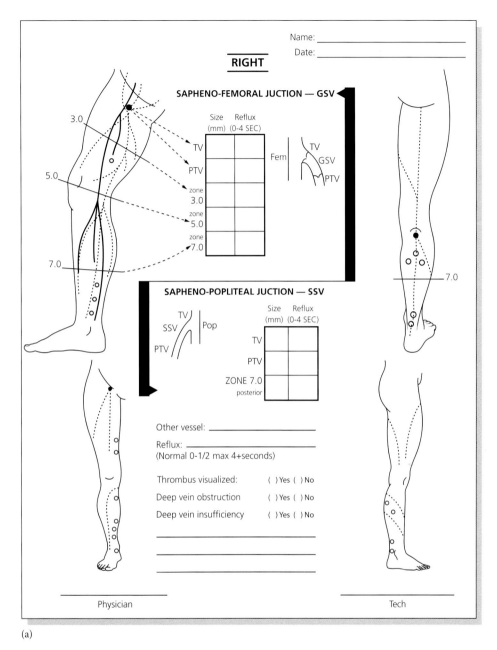

Figure 8.5 Reflux worksheet: (a) right leg and (b) left leg.

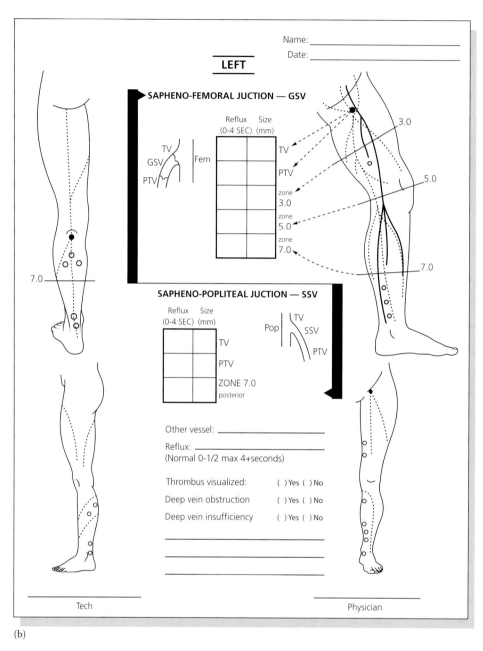

LEFT

Name: _____

Date: _____

▶ **SAPHENO-FEMORAL JUCTION — GSV**

	Reflux (0-4 SEC)	Size (mm)	
TV			TV
GSV PTV	Fem		PTV
			zone 3.0
			zone 5.0
			zone 7.0

3.0

5.0

7.0

7.0

SAPHENO-POPLITEAL JUCTION — SSV

	Reflux (0-4 SEC)	Size (mm)	
			TV
Pop			SSV
			PTV
TV			
PTV			
ZONE 7.0 posterior			

Other vessel: _____

Reflux: _____
(Normal 0-1/2 max 4+seconds)

Thrombus visualized: ( ) Yes ( ) No

Deep vein obstruction   ( ) Yes ( ) No

Deep vein insufficiency   ( ) Yes ( ) No

_____

_____

_____

_____   _____
Tech   Physician

(b)

Figure 8.5 *(Continued)* Reflux worksheet: (a) right leg and (b) left leg.

Figure 8.6 This worksheet shows a left femoral vein deep vein thrombosis (DVT). The key aspects of this document are the notations of the changes in the venous waveforms in the table below – i.e. absence or reduction in phasicity, augmentation, and spontaneity. A key point is noted in that the waveforms from the right common femoral vein (CFV) are normal, suggesting the left-side pathology does not extend into the inferior vena cava (IVC), and reinforcing the importance of always checking the contralateral CFV if performing a unilateral duplex. Additionally, the DVT location is drawn on to the vein map showing its location from the femoral-profunda split to the level of the popliteal.

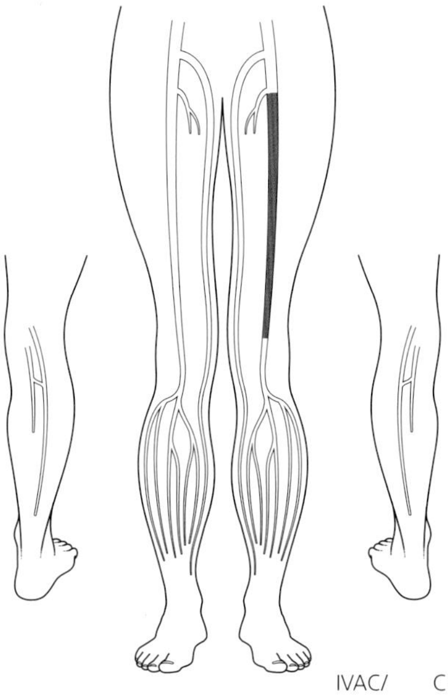

Lower Extremity Venous Duplex

Patient name: _RT DVT — MULTIPLE SITES_ Date: _____

Reffering M.D: _____ Study performed by: _____

Indications: _____ Prior Exam: Date/Result _____

History:

☒ Swelling	☐ CHF	☒ Recent Surgery	☐ Previous Mapping	☐ Pregnancy
☐ Smoking	☐ Prior DVT	☒ Birth Control Pill	☐ Obesity	☒ varicose veins
☐ Chemo/XRT	☐ Malignancy	☐ Hormone Therapy	☐ Anticoagulation	☐ Polycythemia

Hyper-coagulability State: _____

Study ☒ Right ☐ Left ☐ Bilateral

Preliminary Impression

Right

Thrombus - Iliac, Pop, Per
GSV @ SFJ, GSV @ Calf
_____
_____

Left

CFV shows patency
w/ good waveform
_____

Thrombus: Possible
☒ Acute ☒ Chronic ☐ Recanalization

Preliminary Report As Requested

Reviewed by _____ Time _____

Phoned to _____ Time _____

	TLT IVAC/ Iliac	CFV R/L	PFV R/L	SFV R/L	Pop R/L	PTV R/L	Saph R/L
Compressible	—				—		
Spontaneous	—				—		
Phasic	—				—		
Augment	↓				↓		
Partial Comp	✓				✓		
Partial Flow	✓				✓		

_____ Physician

Tech

Figure 8.7 This worksheet shows a right common femoral vein deep vein thrombosis (DVT), with extension into the great saphenous vein, and deep vein thrombosis of the popliteal vein. The key aspects of this document are the notations of the changes in the venous waveforms in the table below – i.e. absence or reduction in phasicity, augmentation, and spontaneity. Again, a key point is noted in that the waveforms from the left common femoral vein (CFV) are normal, suggesting the right-side pathology does not extend into the inferior vena cava (IVC), and reinforcing the importance of always checking the contralateral CFV if performing a unilateral duplex. Additionally, the DVT location is drawn on to the vein map. Showing its location in the CFV extending from the GSV, distal FV, and into the Pop V.

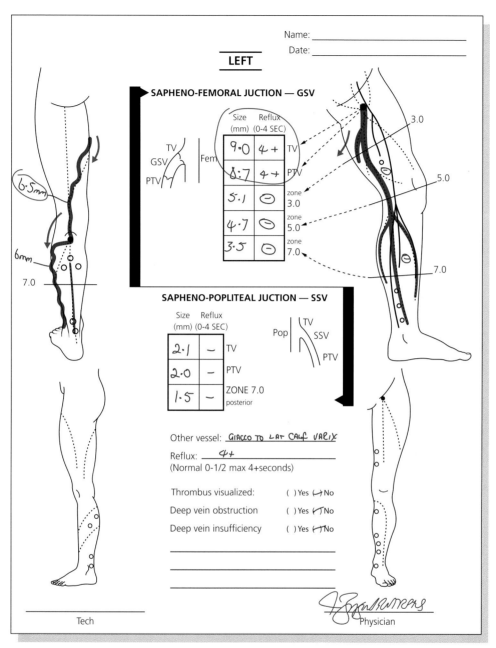

LEFT

Name: _____
Date: _____

SAPHENO-FEMORAL JUCTION — GSV

Size (mm)	Reflux (0-4 SEC)	
9·0	4 +	TV
8·7	4 +	PTV
5·1	⊖	zone 3.0
4·7	⊖	zone 5.0
3·5	⊖	zone 7.0

SAPHENO-POPLITEAL JUCTION — SSV

Size (mm)	Reflux (0-4 SEC)	
2·1	–	TV
2·0	–	PTV
1·5	–	ZONE 7.0 posterior

Other vessel: _GIACCO TO LAT CALF VARIX_

Reflux: ___4+___
(Normal 0-1/2 max 4+seconds)

Thrombus visualized: ( ) Yes (↪)No

Deep vein obstruction   ( ) Yes (↪)No

Deep vein insufficiency   ( ) Yes (↪)No

_____
_____
_____

_____   _____
Tech   Physician

Figure 8.8 This is a left-sided reflux evaluation. This shows incompetence of the saphenofemoral junction (SFJ) that dumps into the posterior accessory, flowing into the Giacomini vein and the varicosities of the lateral posterior calf. A key point is that the great saphenous vein (GSV) below the posterior accessory is normal, without reflux, and, the small saphenous vein (SSV) is normal from the popliteal distally.

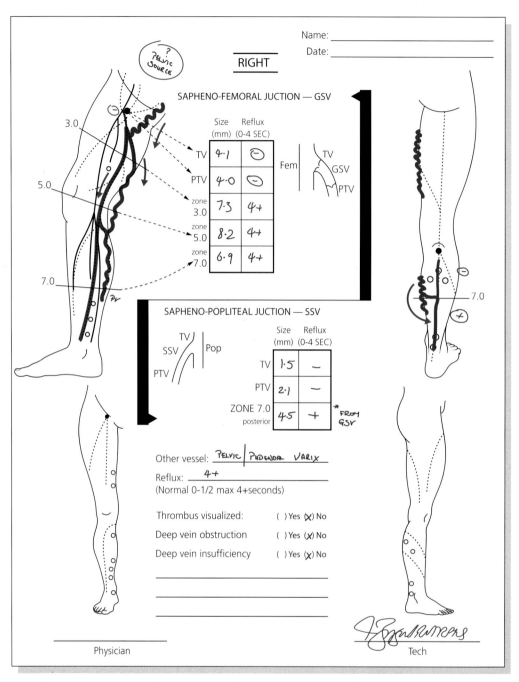

Figure 8.9 This is a right-sided reflux evaluation. There are a few key points noted here. First, the saphenofemoral junction (SFJ) is competent. The source of reflux is a pudendal source. This reflux descends to join the great saphenous vein (GSV) at the point, below the preterminal valve. There is axial reflux down the GSV and into a posterior accessory GSV tributary from the upper thigh along the entire medial aspect of the leg. Also a large posterior varix carries reflux from the medial calf varices to the distal small saphenous vein (SSV), resulting in reflux in the distal SSV. There is also a terminal perforator noted on the medial calf, which appears to be a re-entry site for the superficial venous overload.

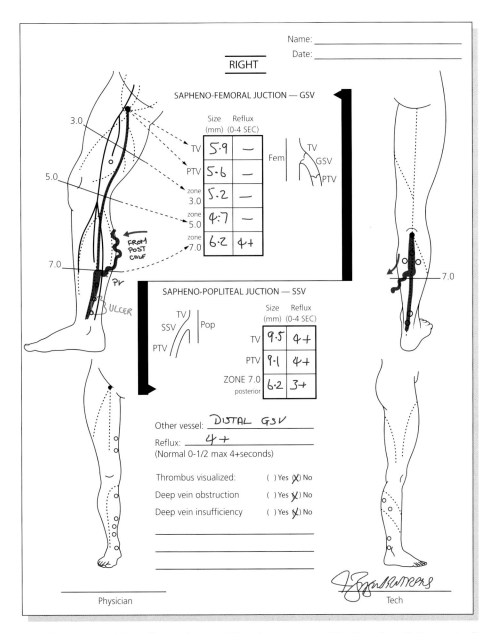

Figure 8.10 This is a right-sided reflux evaluation. There is saphenopopliteal junction dilation and reflux. The reflux is communicated to the medial calf through a varicose complex and dumps into the distal great saphenous vein (GSV) with a dilated perforator and ulcer of the medial malleolous. This demonstrates a 'cross-over' pattern as described by Obermeyer, in which although there is a medial ankle ulceration, the source of reflux is not the saphenofemoral junction (SFJ/GSV), but the small saphenous vein (SSV). In this instance, inaccurate diagnosis with duplex could lead to an ablation of the GSV which does not correct the source of the venous insufficiency.

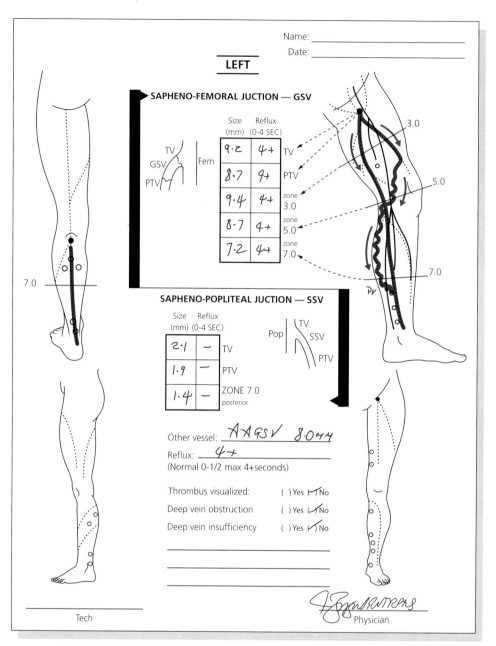

Figure 8.11 Left-sided reflux evaluation. The key finding here is that there is reflux through both the saphenofemoral junction (SFJ) and great saphenous vein (GSV), as well as through the anterior accessory great saphenous vein (AAGSV). The GSV is 8–9 mm, and the AAGSV is 8 mm. If done in a transverse view, following distal compression, no reflux would be seen in the deep system, but reflux would be present in both the GSV and AAGSV. Reflux descends in both of these axial veins, and adequate treatment would involve treatment of both of these veins, as well as the distal manifestations. Also noted is a perforator above the medial ankle, which is most likely a re-entry perforator. The perforator would be best understood if restudied about 90 days after the removal of the GSV and AAGSV overload.

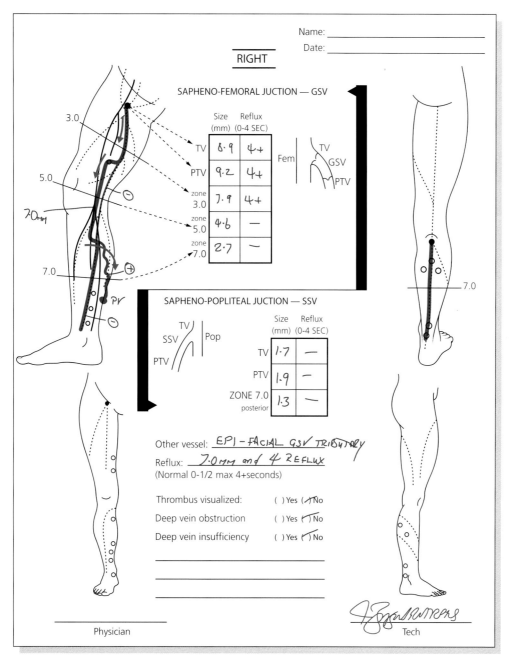

Name: _____
Date: _____

RIGHT

SAPHENO-FEMORAL JUCTION — GSV

	Size (mm)	Reflux (0-4 SEC)
TV	6.9	4+
PTV	9.2	4+
zone 3.0	7.9	4+
zone 5.0	4.6	—
zone 7.0	2.7	~

SAPHENO-POPLITEAL JUCTION — SSV

	Size (mm)	Reflux (0-4 SEC)
TV	1.7	—
PTV	1.9	—
ZONE 7.0 posterior	1.3	—

Other vessel: _EPI – FACIAL GSV TRIBUTARY_

Reflux: _7.0 MM and 4 REFLUX_

(Normal 0-1/2 max 4+seconds)

Thrombus visualized: ( ) Yes (✓) No

Deep vein obstruction   ( ) Yes (✓) No

Deep vein insufficiency   ( ) Yes (✓) No

_____

_____

_____

_____ Physician

Tech

Figure 8.12 Right-sided reflux evaluation. Here, the reflux descends from the saphenofemoral junction (SFJ) and into the proximal great saphenous vein (GSV). However, at about zone 4, the reflux leaves the sheath, entering a GSV epifascial tributary (the so-called 'h' pattern). The GSV below this branch does not show reflux in the distal thigh or lower leg. The reflux from the 'h-vein' crosses over the saphenous at zone 7, and floods reflux into the varices along the posterior arch distribution, with a large terminal perforator noted distally.

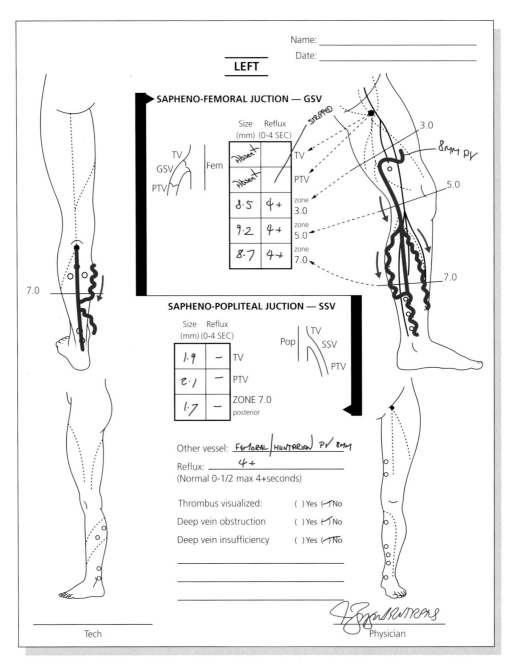

Figure 8.13 Left-sided reflux evaluation. In this patient, previous surgical intervention removed the saphenofemoral junction (SFJ) and proximal great saphenous vein (GSV). A large (8 mm) incompetent perforator dumps reflux from the deep system into a remnant GSV segment in the hunterian canal. The remnant GSV is 8–9 mm with significant reflux along the medial calf, and into the varices of the medial, posterior, and anterior lower leg. This demonstrates how an incomplete initial operative procedure can lead to a significant recurrence.

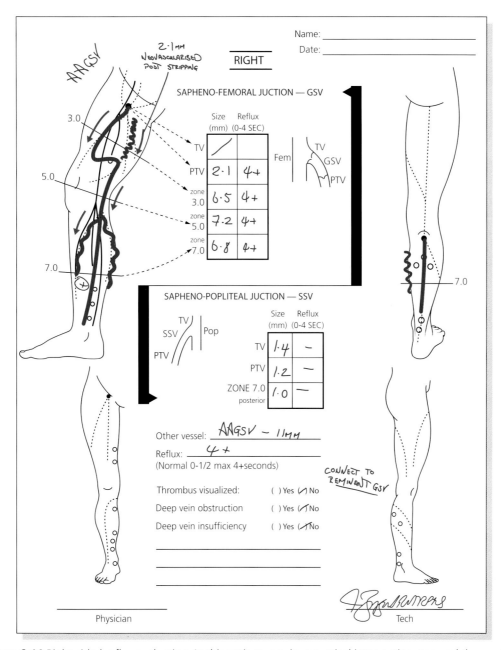

Figure 8.14 Right-sided reflux evaluation. In this patient, previous surgical intervention removed the most proximal segment of the great saphenous vein (GSV). However, there is neovascularization of that segment with a curly-q vein complex from the groin to the mid-thigh. Also, there is incompetence of the AAGSV (11 mm with significant reflux) that rejoins the remnant GSV in the mid to distal thigh to dump additional reflux into the superficial venous system below this point. This too shows recurrence from incomplete treatment – of note, both the AAGSV and the neovascularized segments need to be addressed for adequate treatment of the superficial insufficiency noted in this patient.

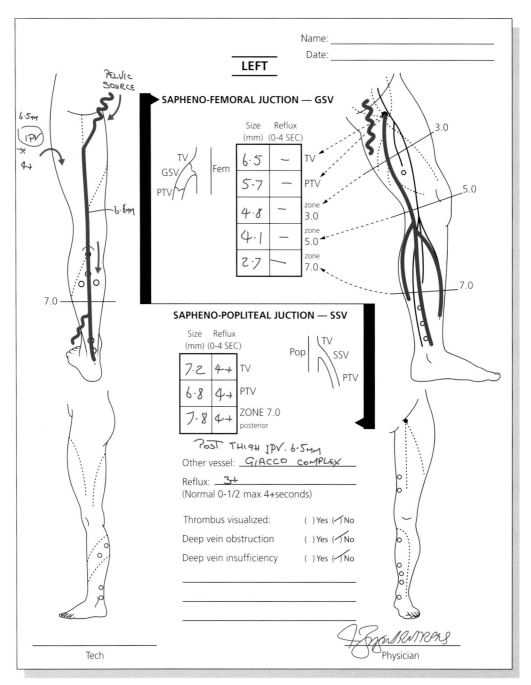

Figure 8.15 Left-sided reflux evaluation. This patient has two sources of reflux. There is a 6.5 mm incompetent perforator of the upper posterior thigh, as well as pelvic source which is dumping reflux down an epifascial pathway in the upper posterior medial thigh to the location of the perforator which joins the cranial extension of the small saphenous vein (SSV) (6.8 mm) and displays reflux into the SSV and its distal varicosities. Of note, the great saphenous vein (GSV) is not involved in this pathology, being normal throughout.

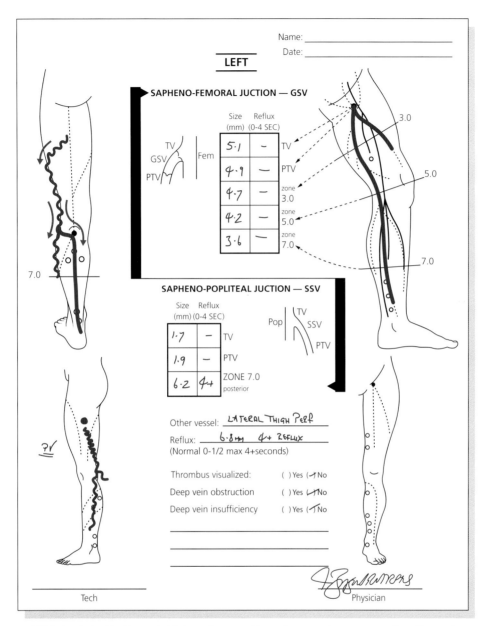

Figure 8.16 This is a left-sided lateral thigh perforator. Above knee perforators are often like an incompetent saphenofemoral junction (SFJ) in that they are exit perforators – and not entry or terminal perforators. In almost all cases, a proximal perforator deserves to be treated. In this case, we have a 6.8 mm lateral thigh perforator. There is 4+ seconds of reflux which descends down the varicose complex of the lateral thigh, dumping into the lateral calf, and also into the upper portion of the small saphenous vein. Although the saphenopopliteal junction (SPJ) is of normal function, and without reflux, below the confluence with the varicose complex, the small saphenous vein (SSV) dilates to 6.2 mm with significant reflux distally.

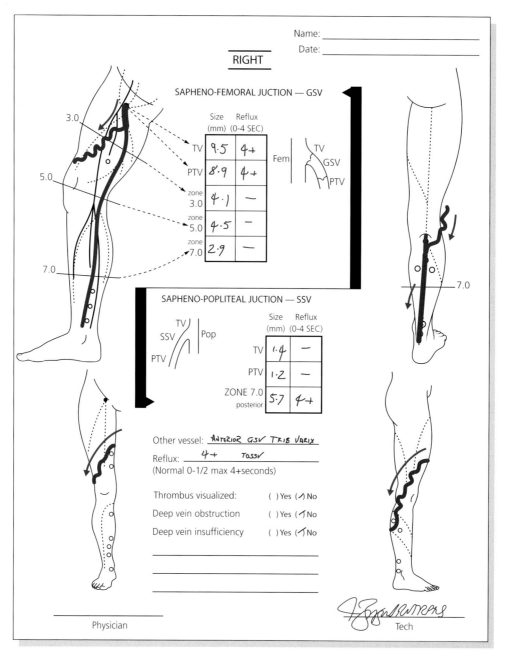

Name: _____

Date: _____

RIGHT

SAPHENO-FEMORAL JUCTION — GSV

	Size (mm)	Reflux (0-4 SEC)
TV	9.5	4+
PTV	8.9	4+
zone 3.0	4.1	—
zone 5.0	4.5	—
zone 7.0	2.9	—

SAPHENO-POPLITEAL JUCTION — SSV

	Size (mm)	Reflux (0-4 SEC)
TV	1.4	—
PTV	1.2	—
ZONE 7.0 posterior	5.7	4+

Other vessel: _ANTERIOR GSV TRIB VARIX_

Reflux: ___4+___ _ToSSV_

(Normal 0-1/2 max 4+seconds)

Thrombus visualized: ( ) Yes (✓) No

Deep vein obstruction   ( ) Yes (✓) No

Deep vein insufficiency   ( ) Yes (✓) No

_____

_____

_____

_____
Physician

_____
Tech

Figure 8.17 This is a right-sided saphenous junction incompetence – with a twist. The incompetence results in reflux in the proximal great saphenous vein (GSV). However, about 10 cm distal to the junction, a large epifascial tributary is noted anterior. The GSV below this is of normal caliber (4–5 mm) and normal function. All of the reflux descends along the anterior epifascial tributary. It dumps into the anterior thigh, the lateral thigh, and then into the proximal small saphenous vein (SSV). The saphenopopliteal junction is normal. This is another example of a crossover pattern as described by Obermeyer – although this is an anterior and lateral pattern, where most are posterior and medial.

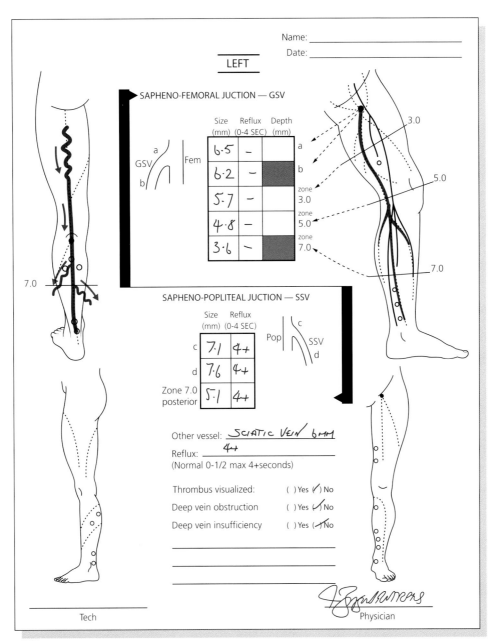

Name: _____

Date: _____

LEFT

SAPHENO-FEMORAL JUCTION — GSV

	Size (mm)	Reflux (0-4 SEC)	Depth (mm)	
a	6·5	–		a
	6·2	–		b
	5·7	–		zone 3.0
	4·8	–		zone 5.0
	3·6	~		zone 7.0

GSV   Fem

3.0

5.0

7.0

7.0

SAPHENO-POPLITEAL JUCTION — SSV

	Size (mm)	Reflux (0-4 SEC)
c	7.1	4+
d	7.6	4+
Zone 7.0 posterior	5.1	4+

Pop   SSV
c
d

Other vessel: _SCIATIC VEIN 6MM_

Reflux: _____4+_____

(Normal 0-1/2 max 4+seconds)

Thrombus visualized: ( ) Yes (✓) No

Deep vein obstruction   ( ) Yes (✓) No

Deep vein insufficiency   ( ) Yes (✓) No

_____

_____

_____

_____
Tech

_____
Physician

Figure 8.18 This shows a varicose complex of the left posterior thigh. The reflux descends along the thigh extension (or cranial extension) of the small saphenous vein (SSV) and into the SSV proper below the knee. Of particular note is the vein wrapped around the sciatic vein, which is of concern in choosing a treatment approach.

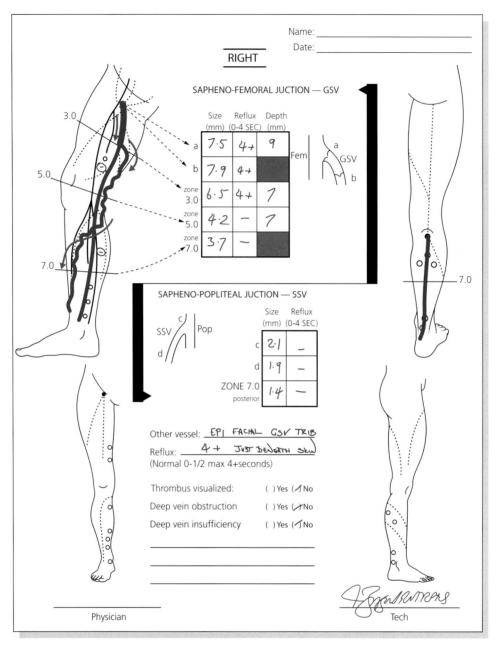

Figure 8.19 A right-sided saphenous incompetence on the depth mapping form. This shows a saphenofemoral junction (SFJ) that is incompetent with gross reflux into the proximal great saphenous vein (GSV). At about zone 3, the reflux leaves the saphenous canal, descending in an epifascial (and axial) GSV tributary. The key here is that the GSV in the sheath (and at a depth of 7 mm) is only about 4 mm without reflux. The epifascial varix maintains a 6–7 mm diameter and is just beneath the skin as far as depth, with 4+ seconds of reflux along the medial thigh. It crosses over the saphenous vein proper below the knee, and feeds the varicose complex of the tibial segment of the leg. Note: The GSV below the knee does not have any reflux.

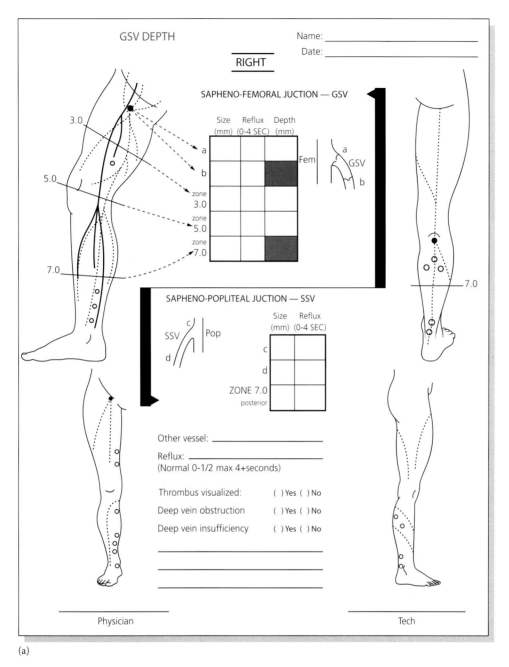

(a)

Figure 8.20 a,b Vein maps with a space to indicate the depth of the great saphenous vein.

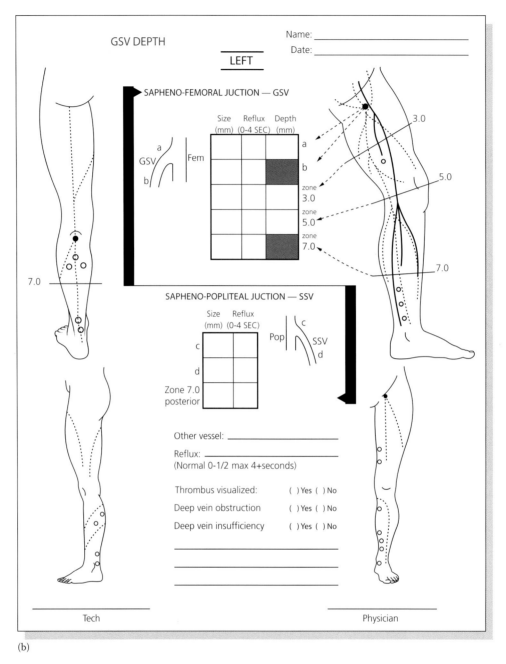

(b)

Figure 8.20 (Continued) a,b Vein maps with a space to indicate the depth of the great saphenous vein.

Vein maps with depth boxes

Figure 8.18 and 8.19 are vein maps that additionally have a 'space' to indicate the depth of the great saphenous vein (GSV) along its course. This is a key factor in endovenous thermal ablation as a certain depth is required as to not injure (burn) the skin with a thermal device. When these devices were first marketed, most would avoid superficial vein treatment due to this concern. With advancing skill and knowledge, a superficial vein can be pushed deeper with perivenous tumescent anesthesia – and this became less of a problem. Figures 8.20 a,b are blank versions of the vein maps with depth boxes as noted. This is especially important to those new to the field as a a reminder of the importance of saphenous depth for a safe ablation procedure and for consideration of not only thermal protection but also the potential for development of a palpable hard cord which may be a suboptimal result.

More recently, the depth measurements were taken out of the diagram, resulting in the versions currently used. However, a sonographer should still note if there is a particular concern with vein depth for procedure-planning purposes on the newer forms.

Conclusion

All too often, when the sonographer or physican sees the anatomy and pathology, they struggle with how to best document and communicate this information. This chapter presents blank worksheets and examples of various pathology with the affiliated documentation as suggested in each situation. Naturally, a fully explanatory dictation should accompany each report with the diagram attached. The practice of having both the dictated report and the vein map diagram to refer to is becoming standard of care in those facilities which specialize in this type of treatment. This pattern is very helpful, communicates information in a simple manner, and should be encouraged and widely adopted.

9

Appendix

This appendix contains a compendium of information which is available on-line from multiple sources. It is intended to be a reference or resource section, leading the interested reader to investigate these other informative sources. Along with a short description, most of these items provide the web address listed as a link for the entire document. Many of these sources have living documents which are updated from time to time, due to the changing nature of medicine, and especially with phlebology. Over the past 10–15 years, the increased interest in this area has had a significant impact on the development of this information.

American College of Phlebology (ACP) – Duplex ultrasound guidelines (**Figure 9.1**)

American College of Phlebology – Scope of practice for sonographers statement (**Figure 9.2**)

American College of Phlebology website: Much more information can be found at www.phlebology.org.

American College of Radiology (ACR) provides a position statement on quality control and improvement, safety, infection control and patient education. This document provides information on aspects of these topics for a well-run and well-documented ultrasound department. More information and the entire document can be found at www.acr.org/SecondaryMainMenuCategories/quality_safety/guidelines/position_statement.aspx.

From the ACR website, a ten-page document 'Ultrasound Accreditation Requirements' with information on personnel qualifications, quality control, accreditation testing, fees and additional information can be found at www.acr.org/accreditation/Ultrasound/Ultrasound_reqs.aspx.

An informative document for anyone performing and interpreting ultrasounds is the ACR Practice Guideline for Performing and Interpreting Diagnostic Ultrasound Examinations, which includes many valuable tips and guidance as delineated fully in the entire document. This can be found at www.acr.org/SecondaryMainMenuCategories/quality_safety/guidelines/us/us_performing_interpreting.aspx.

There is a multiple society document specific to venous ultrasound, ACR-AIUM-SRU Practice Guideline for the Performance of Peripheral Venous Ultrasound Examination which is a resource that anyone performing venous studies should be aware of. This entire document can be found at www.acr.org/SecondaryMainMenuCategories/quality_safety/guidelines/us/us_peripheral_venous.aspx.

American Registry of Diagnostic Medical Sonography (ARDMS). This organization provides for the registered vascular technologist (RVT) sonographer credential. In order to take the test, there are various pathways which are different for sonographers or physicians. These RVT prerequisites include pathways from experience to college ultrasound programs and can be found at www.ardms.org/downloads/prerequisite_chart.pdf.

An additional step in the process for the RVT exam is the preparation and submission of the clinical verification form, which needs to be signed off by a currently credentialed RVT. This document lists the various knowledge areas which need to be demonstrated by the applicant and is available at www.ardms.org/downloads/DVForms?VT/VTDomestic.pdf.

American Institute of Ultrasound in Medicine (AIUM). This organization also provides guidelines for documentation of ultrasound exams and venous protocols specifically. This information can typically be considered for inclusion in a general handbook of procedures and policies for a vascular laboratory, either hospital or office based. This information is available at www.aium.org/publications/guidelines/documentation.pdf and www.aium.org/publications/guidelines/peripheralVenous.pdf.

American Venous Forum (AVF) (www.veinforum.org). The AVF is a great resource for the venous specialist and provides many resources including:

Courses by the AVF. www.veinforum.org/Medical-and-Allied-Health-Professionals/Education.aspx.

Screening Programs of the AVF. www.veinforum.org/Medical-and-Allied-Health-Professionals/AVF-Initiatives/Screening. aspx.

Cardiovascular Credentialing International (CCI) offers the RVS and RPhS ultrasound credentials. The RPhS specifically has a phlebology focus, while the RVS compares to the RVT being a full vascular ultrasound credential. Their website provides a full application booklet for their examinations and can be found at cci-online.org/sites/default/files/2011_App_Book-FINAL.pdf.

Society of Diagnostic Medical Sonography (SDMS). The SDMS has a scope of practice for the ultrasound professional position statement which correlates closely to others listed here and includes a Minimum Entry Level Competence Document for a Diagnostic Ultrasound Professional, Standards for Clinical Practice and Recognition of Sonography Credentialing Programs which can be found at www.sdms.org/positions/scope.asp, www.sdms.org.pdf/nms_dup.pdf, www.sdms.org/positions/clinicalpractice. asp, and www.sdms.org/positions/recognition.asp.

Society of Vascular Ultrasound (SVU). This is the leading society for vascular ultrasound education in the United States. There are several valuable documents available on their website which have to do with topics which include the following

Minimum entry level competence of a sonographer: www.svunet.org/files/positions/SVU Position7AStandardsforAssurance.pdf.

Scope of practice: www.svunet.org/i4a/pages/index.cfm?pageID=3513.

Study performance guidelines for venous insufficiency: www.svunet.org/files/positions/Lower-ExtremityVenousInsufficiency Evaluation. pdf.

Study performance guidelines for deep vein thrombosis: www.svunet.org/files/positions/0608Lower_Extremity_Venou.pdf.

Society of Interventional Radiology (SIR) provides several key documents for clinical practice guidelines, guidelines of quality improvement, position statements on endovenous ablation, endovascular deep vein treatment, a position statement on endovascular pelvic venous insufficiency which can be found at

SIR – Clinical practice guidelines. www.sirweb.org/clinical/cpg/S199.pdf.

SIR – Guidelines for quality improvement program in interventional radiology. www.sirweb.org/clinical/cpg/S203.pdf.

SIR – Position statement on endovenous ablation. www.sirweb.org/clinical/cpg/SIR_venous_ablation_statement_final_Dec03.pdf.

SIR – Chronic cerebrovascular insufficiency CCSVI position statement. www.sirweb.org/clinical/cpg/1520.pdf.

SIR – Joint statement with American Venous Forum on reporting standards for Endovenous Ablation. www.sirweb.org/clinical/cpg/Endovenous_Ablation_for_the_Treatment_of_Venous_Insufficiency.pdf.

SIR – Position statement on endovascular treatment of deep vein thrombosis. www.sirweb.org/clinical/cpg/417.pdf.

SIR – Position statement on endovascular treatment of pelvic venous insufficiency. www.sirweb.org/clinical/cpg/tech25.pdf.

Sound ergonomics is a company that provides a wealth of information on ergonomics, positioning and prevention of musculoskeletal disorders in sonography at their website www.soundergonomics.com/pdf/WRMSDweb.pdf.

Duplex Ultrasound Imaging of Lower Extremity Veins in Chronic Venous Disease, Exclusive of Deep Venous Thrombosis: Guidelines for Performance and Interpretation of Studies

Task force: John Bergan MD, Robert Min MD, Steven Zimmet MD, and Joe Zygmunt Jr RVT

These American College of Phlebology guidelines for lower extremity ultrasound venous imaging describe minimum standards for imaging protocols and reporting, as well as qualifications for those individuals performing and interpreting these studies. The accuracy of the non-invasive venous study depends on the knowledge, skill and experience of the technologist or physician performing the studies, and the knowledge, skill and experience of the physician interpreting the studies.

The ultrasound investigation in patients with chronic venous disease (CVD) is very different from examinations to rule out deep vein thrombosis. Most examinations for CVD are for diagnosis and planning for treatment of venous insufficiency. The information gathered by the duplex investigation has a significant impact on what type of treatment will be most appropriate and therefore recommended. Failure to identify and treat all sources of reflux may result in outright treatment failure. Duplex ultrasound is essential to the performance and ultrasound-guided sclerotherapy. The examination may be used for outcome assessment after treatment.

Indications for Duplex Doppler Ultrasoundstudies in Chronic Venous Disorders

Duplex ultrasound imaging is the most commonly used investigation to evaluate the venous system prior to management of chronic venous disorders of the lower extremities. After a focused history and a physical examination, a request should be made for a duplex ultrasound exam. Duplex ultrasonographic imaging is indicated in patients seeking treatment for primary or recurrent venous insufficiency (varicose veins) and in patients with lower extremity symptoms or signs suggestive of venous disorders.

The duplex ultrasound examination in CVD patients should demonstrate both venous anatomy and function. The following facts should be determined during the standing examination:

1) The location, competency and diameter of the saphenous junctions.
2) The distal extent of reflux in the saphenous veins in the thighs and legs. Recording the saphenous diameter at the mid-thigh and at the knee is desirable.
3) The location of incompetent perforating veins as measured from the floor.
4) Other named and unnamed veins that show reflux or are varicose should be noted.
5) The source of venous hypertension in varices if not from the veins described above.
6) Saphenous veins that are absent, totally occluded, hypoplastic or atretic should be noted.
7) The state of the deep venous system, including valvular competence and evidence of current or previous venous thrombosis.

Qualification to perform and/or interpret duplex ultrasound imaging does not constitute qualification to perform endovenous ablation procedures. Additional training in those techniques is mandatory.

Equipment

Use of appropriate duplex instrumentation, which uses both B-mode imaging and real-time Doppler ultrasound, is required. A color duplex ultrasound instrument is recommended. Imaging probes of 7–15MHz are appropriate for obtaining good quality images of the venous system of the legs. Doppler frequencies of at least 3MHz and hard copy documentation of the examination are recommended. Static images must be archived.

Patient Positioning

Evaluation of the superficial system is best performed on the non-weight-bearing extremity with the patient standing. The supine position is inappropriate for detection of reflux and measurement of vein diameters.

Figure 9.1 ACP Guidelines for diagnostic CVI (reflux) ultra sound studies.

Duplex Ultrasound Imaging of Lower Extremity Veins in Chronic Venous Disease, Exclusive of Deep Venous Thrombosis: Guidelines for Performance and Interpretation of Studies

Definition of Reflux

Reflux determination is considered positive for any reverse (retrograde) flow of greater than 0.5 seconds in the superficial venous sytem, 1.0 second for the femoral or popliteal veins, and 0.35 seconds for perforating veins.

Examination of calf veins may be performed with the patient in either the sitting or standing position. For examination of the tibial and calf vessels, the patient may need to be tilted or the leg dangled over the side of the examination table.

Evaluation of the deep venous system of the thigh may be carried out with the patient supine or in a reverse Trendelenburg position. The flexed leg may be externally rotated for better access to the deep venous circulation. Access to the popliteal vein or posterior calf veins may be performed by way of a posterior approach with the patient in a lateral decubitus position.

Reporting of Results

The report should clearly state the reason for the ultrasound examination. A diagrammatic representation of the findings is highly desirable. A textual report is required. The report should include information about the location of sources of venous reflux, status of the saphenous junctions, function of the saphenous veins and the deep venous system. Inclusion of selected images from the study is recommended. A video recording does not usually form part of the report.

Qualifications

The appropriate use and interpretation of non-invasive venous studies requires knowledge of venous anatomy, physiology, hemodynamics, and the clinical manifestations of venous disease. In addition, knowledge of ultrasound physics, indications for testing, criteria for diagnosis of venous reflux and thrombosis, technical limitations of the study and an understanding of the skills necessary to perform the studies.

Suggested minimum qualifications for the physician performing and/or interpreting studies include the following, which relate chiefly to interpretation of examinations.

- Hold an active medical licence.
- Clinical experience in phlebology or related vascular specialty.
- Training and understanding of venous anatomy, physiology and hemodynamics, ultrasound physics and instrumentation. Evidence of training in residency, fellowship or postgraduate CME course work that includes these items is required. This should include: supervised experience in an approved training program in which non-invasive venous studies are an integral part of the experience with a minimum of 50 cases. Or, in the absence of the formal training during residency or fellowship, the physician should have experience with at least 100 documented cases.
- CME with specific reference to venous disease including imaging should be maintained at a minimum of 15 credit hours every three years.
- Continuing experience is important to maintaining competence; a minimum of 100 examinations per year is recommended to maintain a physician's interpretation skills.
- Regular interaction with a sonographer, if applicable, to ensure continuous quality control and improvement is desirable.

The clinical experience and training above relate primarily to interpretation of studies. Additional skills training by the physician in performing the examinations is required. The physician should perform a minimum of 100 examinations per year in order to maintain performance skills.

- Training in venous anatomy, physiology, hemodynamics, ultrasound physics, and instrumentation. Evidence of formal training in a supervised setting and continuing CME course work, which includes these principles is required.

Figure 9.1 (Continued) ACP Guidelines for diagnostic CVI (reflux) ultra sound studies.

Duplex Ultrasound Imaging of Lower Extremity Veins in Chronic Venous Disease, Exclusive of Deep Venous Thrombosis: Guidelines for Performance and Interpretation of Studies

- Qualification to perform these studies is best demonstrated by certification or eligibility for certification by nationally recognized certifying body, such as the registered vascular technologist (RVT) credential offered by the American Registry of Diagnostic Medical Sonographers (ARDMS) or the registered vascular specialist (RVS) credential offered by Cardiovascular Credentialing International (CCI).
- CME minimum requirements should be 30 hours every three years.

The American College of Phlebology guidelines are largely based on the International Union of Phlebology's consensus documents on duplex ultrasound investigation of veins in chronic venous disease of the lower limbs. The consensus documents, as well as other materials reviewed in forming the ACP guidelines included, but were not limited to:

- Cavezzi A, Labropoulos N, Partsch H *et al.* Duplex ultrasound investigation of the veins in chronic venous disease of the lower limbs – UIP Consensus Document. Part II Basic principles. *European Journal of Vascular and Endovascular Surgery* 2006; **31**: 288–99.
- Coleridge-Smith P, Labropoulos N, Partsch H *et al.* Duplex ultrasound investigation of the veins in chronic venous disease of the lower limbs – UIP Consensus Document. Part I Anatomy. *European Journal of Vascular and Endovascular Surgery* 2006; **31**: 83–92.
- MedPac recommendations of imaging services, statement of executive director, March 2005.
- ACC/ACP/SCAI/SVMB/SVS. Clinical competence statement on vascular medicine and catheter-based peripheral vascular interventions. *Journal of the American College of Cardiology* 2004; **44**: 941–57.
- ACR practice guideline for performing and interpreting diagnostic ultrasound examinations, as revised and amended 2000, effective January 2001.
- Labropoulos N, Tiongson J, Pryor L *et al.* Definition of venous reflux in lower-extremity veins. *Journal of Vascular Surgery* 2003; **38**: 793–8.
- Society of Vascular Technology. Suggested minimum qualification for physicians interpreting non-invasive vascular diagnostic studies. March 1996.
- Foldes M, Blackburn M. Standing versus supine positioning in venous reflux evaluation. *Journal of Vascular Technology* 1991; **15**: 321–4.
- Registered Physician in Vascular Interpretation examination requirements.
- Clinical Privilege White Paper. The Credentialing Resource Centre, Marblehead, MA, USA.
- Zygmunt J. What is new in Duplex scanning of the venous system. *Perspectives in Vascular Surgery and Endovascular Therapy* 2009; **21**: 94–104.

Disclaimer

Adherence to these guidelines will not ensure successful performance or interpretation of imaging studies in every situation. Furthermore, these guidelines should not be deemed inclusive of all proper methods of imaging or exclusive of other protocols reasonably directed to obtain the same results. The physician and patient must make the ultimate judgment regarding the propriety of any performance and interpretation of studies in light of all the circumstances presented by the individual patient.

These guidelines reflect the best available data at the time they were prepared; the results of future research or technology may require alteration of the minimum standards or imaging protocols and reporting as set out in these guidelines.

Figure 9.1 *(Continued)* ACP Guidelines for diagnostic CVI (reflux) ultra sound studies.

American College of Phlebology. Position statement. Scope of Practice for the Diagnostic Ultrasound Professional

Preamble

The purpose of this document is to endorse previously defined 'Scope of Practice for Diagnostic Ultrasound Professionals' statement and to further specify their roles as members of the health care team, acting in the best interest of the patient. This scope of practice is a 'living' document that will evolve as the technology expands.

Definition of the Profession

The diagnostic ultrasound profession is a multispecialty field covering a wide array of sonographic applications with ever increasing specialization. These diverse specialties are distinguished by their use of diagnostic medical ultrasound as a primary technology in their daily work. Certification is considered the standard of practice in ultrasound. Currently licensure is required in two US states. Medicare and many third-party insurance carriers look to individual or laboratory certification as minimum requirements for reimbursement. Individuals who are not yet certified should reference the scope as a professional model and strive to become certified.

   With regard to phlebology, the specialty of 'vascular technology' is of primary mportance and clinical significance for optimal patient care. Credentials in this area include: registered vascular technologist (RVT), registered vascular specialist (RVS) or registered phlebology sonographer (RPhS).

Scope of Practice of the Profession

The diagnostic ultrasound professional is an individual qualified by professional credentialing and academic and clinical experience to provide diagnostic patient care services using ultrasound and related diagnostic procedures. The scope of practice of the diagnostic ultrasound professional includes those procedures, acts and processes permitted by law, for which the individual has received education and clinical experience, and in which he/she has demonstrated competency.

Diagnostic Ultrasound Professionals

1) Perform patient assessments.
2) Acquire and analyze data obtained using ultrasound and related diagnostic technologies.
3) Provide a summary of findings to the physician to aid in patient diagnosis and management.
4) Use independent judgment and systematic problem-solving methods to produce high quality diagnostic information and optimize patient care.

Note that technicians, technologists and therapists do not qualify to 'treat' varicose veins or inject spider veins (CMS-Florida Medicare MAC – Treatment of varicose veins 2/09).

   Medical procedures including injection of medications or performance of endovascular therapeutic procedures are not part of the scope of practice of an ultrasonographer. It should be noted that in some instances sonographers participate side by side with physicians as 'assistants' during some phlebology procedures. However, this is under the direct and immediate supervision of the physician.

   The American College of Phlebology statement is largely based on the 'scope of practice' position statement of the Society of Diagnostic Medical Sonographers, which is also endorsed by these other sonographic organizations:

* American Institute of Ultrasound Medicine
* American Society of Echocardiography (qualified endorsement)
* Canadian Society of Diagnostic Medical Sonographers
* Society for Vascular Ultrasound

This position statement is not intended as legal advice. The ACP suggests that you check your legal counsel or your state governing body regarding the laws, regulations, or policies as these may vary from state to state.

Figure 9.2 ACP Scope of Practice for Sonographers.

Index